Immunologic Fundamentals

IMMUNOLOGIC FUNDAMENTALS

Nancy J. Bigley, Ph.D.

Professor of Microbiology
University of Health Sciences
The Chicago Medical School
Chicago, Illinois

YEAR BOOK MEDICAL PUBLISHERS, INC.
35 East Wacker Drive/Chicago, Illinois

Reprinted, February, 1976

Library of Congress Catalog Card Number: 74-20146

International Standard Book Number: 0-8151-0800-1

To the Memory of
JOHN F. BUCHER

Preface

The basic biologic concepts of immunology are fundamental to the practice of modern medicine. As a scientific discipline immunology includes immunochemistry and immunobiology. Being a biologic science, immunology includes developmental biology, genetics, biochemistry, microbiology, anatomy and medicine. The intact immune system is but one of many regulatory mechanisms functioning in an individual; it aids the individual in adaptation to environmental stimuli. The immune response is an adaptive response to external stimuli (e.g., microorganisms and pollen) as well as internal stimuli (e.g., dead or dying tissue cells, virus-altered cells, and possibly cancer cells). All of the genetic information, including that of the two-limbed immune system, is present in the fertilized ovum. The immune system evolves during embryogenesis; the capacity to recognize normal "self" stimuli is repressed or even destroyed while the ability to respond to foreign and altered "self" stimuli is emerging. The specific aim of this textbook is directed toward presenting the basic concepts of immunology in such a way that the medical student may form a mental image of the functioning immune system. Hopefully, this conceptual framework will serve the student as the basis upon which the rapidly emerging abundance of immunologic information may be placed so that the knowledge is clinically useful.

Acknowledgments

I am appreciative of the counsel, support and assistance of my many colleagues. Among those to whom I am most grateful are Mary M. Carruthers, Raoul Fresco, Mariette G. Gerber, Milton Goldin, Chang Ling Lee, Robert Z. Maigetter, Jeffrey M. Margolis, Walter I. Melnyczenko, James G. Shaffer and Randall A. Smith. To Raoul Fresco, of Mount Sinai Hospital in Chicago, for graciously providing the photo- and electron micrographs, and to Charles S. Welleck, for the care given to the preparation of the line drawings, I extend a special gratitude.

For taking the time to read and criticize very "rough" copy of this manuscript along with their own busy academic schedules, I am most grateful to John M. Slack and John H. Wallace. Initial encouragement from Parker R. Beamer is appreciated.

For the invaluable editorial assistance given me by Tula G. Bucher in the completion of this text and for both the typing skills and patience of Mary C. Staniec throughout the course of the preparation of the manuscript, I shall always be grateful and am at a loss to express my gratitude adequately.

I am grateful for the help and patience of the staff of Year Book Medical Publishers; I am especially appreciative of the support given me throughout the preparation of this text by Kenneth E. Hoppens and of the editorial assistance of Deb McBride.

To my former professors, M. C. Dodd and the late C. E. Heist, I am grateful for the initiation to the field of immunology and for their continued encouragement.

To my students, thank you for being. It is for you that I wrote this textbook (hopefully, to ease the struggle in your comprehension of the subject matter).

Table of Contents

1. **Introduction to Host-Parasite Interactions** 1
   Virulence 1
   The Host as a Favorable Microenvironment 4
   Establishing Virulence and Measurement of Virulence 7
   Dissemination of Microorganisms within the Host 8
   Host Defense Mechanisms 8

2. **Antigens and Immunogens** 13
   Basic Definitions 13
   What Kinds of Substances are Good Immunogens? 13
   Natural Biologic Substances 13
   Artificial and Synthetic Immunogens 14
   Antigenic Determinant, Valence and Immunodominant Group 16
   Immunization and the Immune Response 17
   Genetic Capacity of the Individual Being Immunized . . . 17
   Immunization versus Immunologic Unresponsiveness and
   Antigen Dose 18
   Chemical Nature and Physical State of Antigen and Antigen
   Processing 20
   Adjuvants 22
   Route of Injection 23
   Antigens and the Immune Response 24
   Exogenous Microbial Antigens 25
   Endogenous Antigens 27

3. **Immunoglobulins** 37
   Immunoglobulins 37
   Structure and Properties of Immunoglobulins 37
   Allotypic Markers of Human Immunoglobulins 45
   Theories of Antibody Formation 46
   Antibody Production 48

ix

Immunoglobulin Levels 55
Biologic Functions of Human Immunoglobulins 58
Pathologic Counterparts of Human Immunoglobulins 61
   Multiple Myelomas 61
   H Chain Diseases 63
   Other Immunoglobulin Abnormalities 66

4. Complement 69
   Activation of Classic Complement Pathway 69
   Complement-Fixation Test 71
   Biologic Significance 72
   The Alternate Complement Pathway 73
   Interrelation of Three Host Cascade Systems 75
   Complement Deficiencies 77

5. Serology: Antigen-Antibody Interactions in Vitro 80
   Characteristics of the Union of Antibody and Antigen 80
   Nature of the Forces Which Bind Antigen and Antibody . . . 80
   Specificity of Antigen-Antibody Interactions 82
   In Vitro Reactions 83
   Titer 84
   Applications of Serologic Tests in Diagnosis 84
   Immune Precipitation Reactions 87
   Variations of the Precipitin Test 87
   The Agglutination Reaction 94
   Complement Fixation 96
   Tissue Typing 96
   Immunocytoadherence: Mixed Cell Agglutination Reactions or
      Rosette Tests 97

6. Cell-Mediated Immunity 99
   Lymphokines 100
   T Cell System 102
   Assays of T Cell Function 103
   Antigen-Specific T Cell Receptors 104
   Transferability of CMI 104
   Induction of Cell-Mediated Immunity 105
   Cell-Mediated Immune Responses In Vivo 105

7. Biology of the Immune Response 108
   Phylogeny 108

Ontogeny. 109
Thymic Humoral Factor 113
T Cell Receptors and Rosette-Forming Cells 114
Lymphocyte Surface Markers 114
    Mouse Cell Markers 114
    Human Cell Markers 115
Nutrition and the Immune Response. 116
Functioning Immunoresponsiveness. 116
Two-Signal Model of Induction of Immune Responses 119
Mobility of Lymphocyte Surface Antigens and Receptors . . . 121
Cellular Interactions 124
Immunologic Deficiency Diseases 125
    Primary Immunodeficiency Diseases 125
    Secondary Immune Deficiency States. 129

8. Host-Parasite Interactions and Protective Host Immunity 140
    Localization and Persistence of Microorganisms Within the
        Host 140
    Microbial Virulence Factors 146
    Protective Host Immunity 148

9. Mechanisms of Immunologic Injury 156
    Type I—Anaphylactic Type Injury 156
    Type II—Cytotoxic Type Injury 160
        Immune Cytolysis of Erythrocytes 160
        Antibody-Mediated Cytotoxicity of Other Cells 163
    Type III—Immune Complex-Mediated Injury 164
    Type IV—Cell Mediated (Delayed Type Hypersensitivity)
        Injury 169
    Antibody-Mediated Stimulation as a Mechanism of Immune
        Injury 171

10. Autoimmunity 174
    Possible Etiologic Mechanisms of Autoimmune Disease . . . 176
    Microbial Agents as Inducers of Autoimmunity 177
    Slow Viruses and Autoimmunity 178
    Drug-Induced Autoimmunity 183

11. Tumor and Allograft Immunity 187
    Host Responses to Tissue Antigens 187
    Host Reactions to Allografted Tissues 188

Possible Interrelationships Between Oncogenesis and Host
Immune Systems 190

The Fetus as an Allograft? 192

HL-A Antigens and Mixed Leukocyte Culture (MLC) Antigens
Used in Tissue Typing 193

β_2 Microglobulin, HL-A System and Lymphocyte Receptors . . 194

12. Manipulations of the Immune Response 197

Vaccination 197

Types of Vaccines Currently in Use 197

Virus Vaccines 197

Bacterial Vaccines 201

Vaccination Regimens and Considerations 204

Biologic Manipulations of the Immune Response
Suppression of Antibody Production by 7S (IgG) 208

Desensitization 208

Transfusions 209

"Transfusion" of Passive Immunity 209

Experimental Manipulations of Immune Response 211

Antilymphocyte Sera 211

Using Antigen as a Specific Probe and Cytotoxic Agents for
Destruction of Antigen-Reactive Cells to Prevent
Sensitization 212

Nonspecific Macrophage Activation 212

Use of Bacterial Products Against Malignant Disease 212

Physical and Chemical Manipulations of the
Immune Response 213

Physical Immunosuppressive Agents (X-Irradiation) 213

Chemical Immunosuppressive Agents 213

Cytotoxic Chemotherapeutic Immunosuppressive Agents . . . 214

Index 219

1 / Introduction to Host-Parasite Interactions

Host-parasite interactions are intimate cellular and even molecular (e.g., virus parasitisms) symbiotic relationships. Simply stated, *symbiosis* is the living together or close association of two dissimilar organisms. The normal microbial flora (microflora) of a human or animal host are considered as *commensals* and the relationship is termed *commensalism,* a relationship which is beneficial to the microorganism and (usually) not harmful to the host. Under certain conditions, the normal microflora may enter into a parasitic relationship with the host. In *parasitism,* the host is injured and the parasite is benefited.

VIRULENCE

Although the term virulence is generally used in describing the pathogenicity (capacity to produce disease) of a given microorganism, it actually describes the degree of pathogenicity of a specific microorganism in an individual host and is the result of the interaction between host and parasite. Some microorganisms possess the ability to invade the host. This capacity is referred to as *aggressin activity.* For example, encapsulated bacteria such as *Diplococcus pneumoniae* are able to resist ingestion by host phagocytes and thereby gain a temporal advantage in that they can multiply. Microorganisms that secrete toxic substances which are injurious to the host and its defense mechanisms gain an advantage in that they, too, can multiply without host interference long enough to produce an infection. Examples of this latter situation are seen in infections initiated by certain strains of group A, beta hemolytic *Streptococcus pyogenes* and strains of pathogenic *Staphylococcus aureus* in which host phagocytes are destroyed by toxic molecules elaborated by the bacteria.

Microorganisms which lack invasive properties may gain entrance into the host by accident. The clostridia, lacking aggressin activity, lead a saprophytic existence in the soil and are also present in the gastrointestinal tract of man and animals. Certain of the clostridia or their endospores enter human or animal tissues via a wound or trauma. Tetanus (induced by *Clostridium tetani*) and gas gangrene (induced by several members of the genus Clostridium; e.g., *C. perfringens*) are disease processes in which a puncture wound or traumatized area of tissue is contaminated with soil and/or excrement. The strictly anaerobic environment essential for clostridial growth is thought to be initiated by the traumatic injury with resultant host cell necrosis and accumulation of injurious lactic acid. Aerobic microorganisms present in the wound then utilize the remaining available oxygen, thereby establishing an anaerobic crypt. Once anaerobic conditions are achieved the clostridial growth is initiated and a by-product of that growth is the excretion of potent exotoxins. Although these clostridial infections are usually localized at the site of injury, the toxins are able to gain entrance into the circulation and other tissues with serious consequences to the host. Another example of a localized infection and generalized toxemia is diphtheria. *Corynebacterium diphtheriae* initiates its focus of infection usually in the nasopharynx, but can, in rare instances, set up a focal infection at the site of a wound (wound diphtheria) with subsequent excretion of its exotoxin into the host. It is of interest here to note that the pseudomembrane characteristic of the diphtheritic lesion is the result of the host's inflammatory response to the bacteria and its toxic products. Although not included in the scope of this text, the process whereby *C. diphtheriae* and several strains of *Clostridium botulinum* gain the capacity to synthesize and secrete their potent exotoxins is under the genetic control of bacteriophage deoxyribonucleic acid (DNA). This process is termed phage or lysogenic conversion. Without a specific bacteriophage, each of these bacteria would be harmless. This is a peculiar type of synergism in which our parasites have their own molecular parasites.

Another way in which noninvasive microbial parasites gain entrance into human and animal hosts is through the bite of an insect or arthropod vector. Many exotic diseases are transmitted in this manner. The viral encephalitides are transmitted from animal to man and to other animals by insect and arthropod vectors. Yellow fever virus is transmitted by the female *Aedes aegypti* mosquito. Today, all of the virus parasites transmitted to man by insects (mainly mosquitoes) or arthropods such as ticks are classified as *arboviruses* (arthropod-borne viruses). All arboviruses appear capable of replicating in their vectors. Such infected vectors remain infected and asymptomatic during their lifespan. Most rickettsial diseases are vector-borne to man. Rickettsiae thrive selectively in the endothelial cells of the blood vessels, the sites at which they are deposited and from which they disseminate to other endothelial cells. The plague bacillus, *Yersinia pestis,* is vector-borne to man by either rat flea or the human louse. The plague bacillus resides endemically in rodent hosts of South and Central America and in the southwestern United States as do appropriate vectors. Numerous protozoan diseases are vector-borne to man. Certain pathogenic protozoa undergo several asexual and sexual reproductive cycles in different host species; unfortunately, man can serve as one of these hosts. Undoubtedly, the most dramatic protozoan disease in humans is malaria. In malaria, man may serve as the host of the asexual life cycle (shizogony) of the Plasmodium species; i.e., man is their intermediate host. The sexual phase of the life cycle (sporogony) takes place in certain female mosquitoes, i.e., the definitive host.

For infectious diseases to occur, microorganisms must penetrate the host barriers (the intact skin, conjunctiva or mucous membranes). These barriers are routes or portals of microbial entry into the host. Except for vector-borne transmission, most microorganisms are transmitted either directly (by inhalation, ingestion or venereally) or indirectly through fomites (contaminated inanimate objects) between the diseased and susceptible hosts.

If the microbial invader is a virus it must survive the host microenvironment successfully until it reaches suitable host cells to which it may gain entrance and within which it may either survive or replicate itself. If the microbial invader is a procaryotic (e.g., bacteria) or eucaryotic (e.g., fungi and protozoa) microorganism, it, too, must survive long enough to multiply to numbers sufficient to cause disease (alteration of structure and/or function) in the host. In this survival of the invading parasite on the skin, conjunctiva or mucous membrane surfaces of the host, it must compete with the resident microflora for space and nutrients. Within hours following birth, the human infant may be colonized by staphylococci and within days to weeks by gram-negative enteric bacilli (e.g., *Escherichia coli*). The individual species which comprise the resident microflora appear stable over a period of time. For example, the resident staphylococcal microflora of the skin and mucous membranes, especially that of the anterior nares, in humans has been observed to aid in the prevention of colonization by other strains of staphylococcus. In mice, the presence of bacteroides in the gut appears to afford protection against experimental salmonellosis. The normal microflora thus establish a balance for space and nutrients among themselves and an equilibrium with their individual host. Certain antibiotics may disrupt the balance among the members of an individual's microflora present on the mucous membranes of the mouth, gastrointestinal tract and vagina. Consequently, susceptible bacteria are temporarily eradicated and the fungal flora (not susceptible to the antibacterial agents) overgrow, and, in turn, cause disease. Reestablishment of the balance among the normal microflora eventually occurs.

THE HOST AS A FAVORABLE MICROENVIRONMENT

The host tissues supply the necessary optimal environment (e.g., nutrients, oxygen, carbon dioxide, pH, etc.) for microbial growth. Most bacterial pathogens are facultative anaerobes in their oxygen requirement and grow optimally at 37° C in the human host. Rather unique types of infection are produced by several species of mycobacteria whose optimal temperatures of growth are much less than 37° C. *Mycobacterium ulcerans* (grows slowly in primary culture at 30–33° C and will not grow at 37° C) and *Mycobacterium balnei* (also known as *Mycobacterium marinum*; grows at 31° C and not 37° C) only produce skin infections and ulcerations in areas on the host where the temperature is less than 37° C, e.g., the extremities such as the toes, nose, fingers, elbows, knees and legs. The latter microorganism (*M. balnei* or *M. marinum*), originally isolated from saltwater fish, has produced sporadic epidemics and involved individuals who swam in either saltwater or fresh water. There is evidence that *M. leprae* also grow optimally at temperatures less than 37° C.

It has been ingeniously demonstrated that the host serves as a rich source of essential nutrients for microbial parasites. Experiments with nutritional auxotrophs of pathogenic bacteria illustrate the significance of essential nutrients being present in the host to support the growth of certain bacterial pathogens. When these nutritional auxotrophs were injected into mice, no disease ensued. But, when the auxotroph was injected and the nutrient or metabolite required by it was simultaneously injected into, and in some instances fed to, the mice, then the bacteria multiplied and disease became evident. The Brucella species seem to be stimulated by polyerythritol, which is present in high amounts in fetal calves. *D. pneumoniae* lacks a catalase system and readily dies out and autolyzes in broth culture. Yet its natural host, the human, supplies the catalase that this bacterium requires for the inactivation of peroxides generated during its metabolism so that it may multiply and survive in the host.

Normal microflora may cause disease if they change their locale or habitat within the host or if the host's resistance is lowered (a compromised host). With regard to change of locale within the host,

Neisseria meningitidis is part of the normal flora of the nasopharynx of certain humans, but when it gains entrance in some manner into the central nervous system and/or circulation (see "endotoxin shock," Chapter 4) it can produce a rapidly fatal disease. *E. coli* is a normal inhabitant of the gastrointestinal tract of humans, but in the urinary bladder produces cystitis. Since the advent of the use of antibiotics and the accompanying widespread genetic exchanges of drug resistances among the enteric bacilli (Escherichia, Salmonella, Shigella, etc.), an increased incidence of aspiration pneumonia due to *E. coli* has occurred. Dental manipulations may be responsible for the entrance of microorganisms into the blood (bacteremia) and the relocalization within the host.

As examples of lowered host resistance and subsequent disease by normal microflora, none are more intriguing than the bacterial pneumonias which are sequelae to influenza virus infection usually occurring in certain debilitated or aging individuals. Among the normal microflora of the upper respiratory tract in some humans are types of *D. pneumoniae* or *Hemophilus influenzae*. Both of these bacteria are encapsulated pathogens and presumably are held in check normally by a combination of secretory antibody which enhances their ingestion by phagocytes in the mucous secretions (see Chapters 3 and 8). When the influenza virus is the primary infecting agent, the cells of the lung are heavily invaded and replicate virus. Although not killed, the host phagocytes may be seriously and temporarily maimed in their ability to generate energy from glucose. From in vitro studies the glycolytic pathway of such phagocytes was shown to be 90% inhibited by influenza virus. The action of the virus seemed to inhibit at the level of the phosphohexose isomerase; neither glucose nor glucose-6-phosphate was metabolized. If this occurs in vivo, then a likely explanation exists for the occurrence of secondary bacterial pneumonias seen in the wake of influenza epidemics. Similarly, *S. aureus* or beta hemolytic streptococci also may be the bacterial agent in these secondary pneumonias.

In general, the relationship between host malnutrition and infection is synergistic. Infections are more likely to produce more serious consequences in persons who are malnourished, and, in turn, infections have the capacity to convert borderline nutritional deficiencies into severe malnutrition. Occasionally, the undernourished host provides an antagonistic environment for certain viral and protozoan parasites. (Perhaps this is seen because viruses and some protozoan parasites reside inside host cells. If the host is severely malnourished, its cells are possibly deprived of certain essential nutrients and they, in turn, would serve as a poor microenvironment for the replication of viruses or growth of protozoa.) Severe nutritional deficiency interferes with host functions (e.g., the integrity of the skin and mucous membrane barriers, the production of body fluids and enzymes antagonistic to microorganisms, phagocytic functions, antibody formation, and alterations in intestinal microflora).

A synergism among members of the normal microflora may produce disease in the human, usually in the oral cavity. This disease is called fusospirochetosis (Vincent's angina or "trench mouth"). The symbionts are usually normal microflora of the gingiva. The fusiform bacilli (Fusobacterium species) and the spirochetes (*Borrelia buccales, Borrelia vincentii, Treponema microdentium, Treponema mucosum,* and Bacteroides species) increase in number when local host resistance is reduced by trauma or vitamin deficiency. Other species of bacteria apparently are involved as symbionts in this synergism. For example, a Vibrio species in combination with an anaerobic species of streptococci and the fusiform-shaped *T. microdentium* are capable of reproducing this disease in guinea pigs. For infection to occur the proper microbial symbionts must be present in the host. Some evidence exists that a nutritional dependence occurs in which a by-product of one bacterium is an essential growth factor for another symbiont. It is extremely difficult to satisfy the cultural requirements in vitro of many of the contributory bacteria, especially the spirochetes. For example, the spirochete *Bacteroides melaninogenicus* cannot grow in the oral cavity without a vitamin K-like naphthaquinone supplied by diphtheroids. Also, anaerobic conditions, e.g., tissue trauma, must be established for growth of the symbionts. Fusospirochetal symbionts may serve as either primary or secondary invaders in infectious processes involving the upper and lower respiratory tracts, and, on occasion, even involve the skin, the genital areas and the gastrointestinal tract of man. In rare instances, metastases from local lesions may infect any tissue of the body. One of the host's major defense mechanisms against infection by anaerobes is the normal oxidation-reduction potential (Eh = +120 millivolts) of most normal human tissues. When lowering of the redox potential occurs, even in mouth and lungs, anaerobes may multiply. The lowering of tissue redox potentials may result from necrosis, impaired blood supply and prior growth of facultative anaerobes in a wound. The effectiveness of phagocytosis by polymorphonuclear neutrophils and other granulocytes is severely impaired by anaerobic environments.

Even the formation of dental caries is the result of attack by members of the normal microflora. Microorganisms which can both withstand acid environments (aciduric) and ferment carbohydrates to generate acid (acidogenic) are involved in the initiation of caries formation. Yeast and three types of bacteria (streptococci, staphylococci and lactobacilli) are implicated. These microorganisms are present in the dental plaques which form on the enamel surface of teeth and generate the acid which is responsible for the demineralization of the enamel.

ESTABLISHING VIRULENCE AND MEASUREMENT OF VIRULENCE

Virulence of a given microorganism is the result of the host-parasite interaction. Early in the study of microbial disease, Koch established a set of criteria (*Koch's Postulates*) against which a specific microorganism was tested to *prove that the microorganism being examined was the actual etiologic agent of a specific infectious disease.* Koch's Postulates are as follows: that a specific microorganism must be isolated from all individuals with a specific infectious disease; that the microorganism be grown in pure culture; that the pure culture isolate be injected into a second susceptible host; that the same disease be reproduced in the second host from which the same microorganism is isolated and grown in pure culture.

Even today it is not possible to fulfill Koch's criteria for every microbial pathogen. For example, the obligately parasitic bacterial agents of syphilis (*Treponema pallidum*) and leprosy (*M. leprae*) cannot be cultivated in laboratory media following inoculation with material from human lesions.

Even though material from human syphilitic lesions injected into rabbit scrotal tissue may induce a local infection in the rabbit, there is doubt whether the rabbit-grown spirochetes are pathogenic for man. In addition, the growth of these spirochetes in the rabbit does not result in a disease comparable to human syphilis. It has only been in recent years, with improvements in enrichment of culture media and incubation environments, that the virulent form of *Neisseria gonorrhea* was even cultivated. Under these improved conditions, four colony types may be observed. Colonies designated as types 1 and 2 maintain virulence for the human and types 3 and 4 are avirulent.

For the measurement of virulence of a specific microorganism (whether virulence is the result of invasiveness, toxigenicity or a combination of these), standardized procedures are sought. For example, a standard susceptible animal host (age, weight, sex, etc.) is used. A standard route of inoculation, a standard time interval, and a standard endpoint criterion (death or symptoms) are used. The measure is usually expressed in terms of a median dose (of bacteria or toxin) that will kill 50% of the animals inoculated within a stated time period. The number of bacteria which may accomplish this is referred to as a Lethal Dose$_{50}$ (LD$_{50}$).

Virulence can be measured more accurately by establishing LD$_{50}$ dose levels than by measuring the dose which will kill 100% of the inoculated group.

DISSEMINATION OF MICROORGANISMS WITHIN THE HOST

Once the integrity of the host barriers is damaged, microorganisms may be disseminated by the blood stream, by the lymphatic system, within phagocytic cells, by continuity (continuous spreading of the infectious agent within the same tissue or organ) and by contiguity (contiguous dissemination by contamination of an organ or tissue contiguous (next) to the infected organ or tissue). *Mycobacterium tuberculosis* may be spread within the body by any or all of these means. Classically, the mere presence of bacteria in the blood is referred to as a *bacteremia*. Bacteremias ("bacterial showers") have been claimed to occur in healthy individuals periodically without ensuing disease. The presence of viruses in the blood stream is referred to as a *viremia*. The term *septicemia* is employed to describe the process in which microorganisms (usually bacteria) are present and actively metabolizing, multiplying and excreting toxic products in the blood stream.

HOST DEFENSE MECHANISMS

Basically, the three main lines of host defense against microorganisms consist of: the barrier effect of skin, conjunctiva and mucous membranes; the inflammatory response and phagocytosis; and the specific immune response.

The *host barriers* are classified as three anatomically distinct areas. The healthy intact skin is a barrier difficult for microorganisms to penetrate. However, the skin surface does support microbial growth. The fibrous protein keratin comprises the superficial cutaneous layer beneath which are the epidermal cells that die in the process of synthesizing keratin. The sweat glands of the skin provide a weak saline solution and small amounts of nitrogenous nutrient for microorganisms. Hair follicles in the skin exude sebum which is manufactured by the sebaceous glands. Sebum provides lipids and unsaturated fatty acids for microorganisms. Dermatophytes (skin fungi) are keratolytic and thereby contribute amino acids for microbial growth. Carbohydrates and vitamins are less abundant in the skin and its secretions but adequate amounts of each are present for microbial growth. For the most part, the skin is slightly acid and its temperature and water content are suitable for microorganisms. The human skin microflora consist of both aerobic and anaerobic gram-positive microorganisms even though some anerobic gram-negative microorganisms may inhabit the sebaceous glands. Finegold and associates have found a ratio of 10 anaerobic bacteria to every aerobic bacterium in the human skin. The predominant anaerobic skin bacterial flora are diphtheroids (propionibacterium) and gram-positive cocci.

Although the conjunctival membrane is anatomically distinct from mucous membranes, it functionally bears some similarity. Tears contribute to a bathing action of the conjunctiva; antibody (IgA, see Chapter 3) and lysozyme may be found in tears. In comparison to the skin, the membrane surfaces of the host are more easily penetrated by microorganisms. The conjunctiva and mucous membranes of the nasopharynx, respiratory tract, urogenital tracts and gastrointestinal tract serve as significant portals of entry for numerous microbial parasites. As indicated, the secretions of these membranes contain antibody and lysozyme (muramidase), an effective antibacterial substance active against most gram-positive bacteria (except *S. aureus* in which the lysozyme-susceptible site in the cell wall is structurally blocked from lysozyme attack). Mechanical factors contribute to the membrane integrity. For example, the washing action of secretions tends to repel microorganisms; microbial agents may be trapped by mucus-coated hairs in the anterior vestibule of the nose; the membrane surfaces are protected by their adherent mucus covering, the expulsive forces of sneezing and coughing, ciliary action of mucous membranes in the respiratory tract, and the cleansing of the urethra by the flow of urine. Various chemical factors at different mucous membrane sites exhibit effective antimicrobial action. The acidity of the stomach preserves the usual sterility of the stomach. (Microorganisms within food particles or protected by ingested protein may pass through the stomach into the intestinal tract in viable form.) In pernicious anemia with hypochlorhydria, a heavy microbial colonization of the gastric mucosa occurs. Little is yet known of the role of the normal microflora of the human intestinal tract in host nutrition and physiology. Vitamin K is synthesized by *E. coli,* a facultative anaerobe, and by *Bacteroides fragilis,* an anaerobe. While equal numbers of aerobes and anaerobes are present in the mouth, in the colon the ratio of the numbers of *B.*

fragilis to *E. coli* is 1000:1. In the postpubertal and premenopausal female, the vagina is rich in glycogen deposits stimulated by estrin. This environment favors the growth of a Lactobacillus species (Döderlein's bacillus) which produces acid. In prepubertal and postmenopausal women, the vaginal flora differs and is composed of diphtheroides (Corynebacterium species), enterococci (Streptococcus group D) and *Staphylococcus epidermidis* (or *Staphylococcus albus*). *Candida albicans* (a fungus) can induce in the latter group of females as well as in pregnant women and diabetics either vaginitis or vulvovaginitis. Candidiasis of the oral mucous membranes (thrush) occurs in infants contaminated during passage through the birth canal and in debilitated elderly individuals. Lysozyme is present not only in tears but also in nasal secretions and saliva. The polyamine spermine, present in semen and seminal fluids, is bactericidal to a wide range of pathogenic bacteria. The secretory antibody system (IgA) is associated with host resistance throughout the mucous membrane surfaces of the human.

Once the surface of the intact barrier is injured or irritated, microorganisms may penetrate deeper into the host. In the subepithelial connective tissue which is the usual site of primary lodgment of the invader, phagocytes (termed wandering macrophages, histiocytes or monocytes of the reticuloendothelial system) are present. These cells promptly ingest a portion of the invading microorganisms. Those microbes that escape evoke an inflammatory response. The injury is a signal to mobilize the host's inflammatory response to the site of insult.

In brief, dilation of the surrounding blood vessels occurs. Vascular permeability increases permitting the escape of blood plasma, leukocytes and even a few erythrocytes. The granulocytic white blood cells (polymorphonuclear neutrophils or PMNs) pass between endothelial cells of the blood vessel to the site of injury. This process is termed *diapedesis.* In the early phase of the inflammatory response, PMNs are the predominant phagocytic cell. Thus, the early phase of inflammation is called the granulocytic phase. However, after a few hours but certainly within 12 hours, monocytic phagocytes enter the injured site and eventually are the predominate phagocyte. The later phase of an inflammatory response is called the monocytic phase. Present in the plasma exudate are serum, immunoglobulins (mainly IgG, IgM and serum IgA), complement and fibrinogen. If antibody activity to invading microorganisms is present in the exudate, the antibody may coat the bacterial surface and thereby facilitate ingestion by the phagocytes. Fibrin is deposited in the host's attempt to wall off the injured site.

If the invaders are not contained at the initial site of the inflammatory response, the local lesion persists and the microorganisms are transported via the lymphatics to the draining lymph nodes. Here, a repeat of the "inflammatory treatment" ensues. Here also is the site where immune responses are initiated. The reticuloendothelial macrophages phagocytize bacteria washed in from afferent lymphatics. Those bacteria remaining may stimulate an acute inflammation of the lymphatics (lymphadenitis) which, in turn, greatly augments the filtering capacity of the lymph nodes. The sinus channels are jammed with PMNs and eventually monocytes. If, after all of these events, viable microorganisms still exist, some may escape, penetrate the regional lymph node, enter the thoracic duct and then the blood stream. In the blood stream, the granulocytes and monocytes are phagocytic. There are additional reticuloendothelial phagocytes lining the vascular sinusoids of organs such as liver and spleen through which the blood circulates. Microorganisms disseminated in this way may eventually be destroyed, but, in the process, may relocalize and invade in virtually any part of the body.

The specific immune responses are the third line of host defense against microbial attack. Before discussing the terminology and significance of microbial immunology, it must be realized that: (1) the ultimate host "victory" over microbial invaders is the successful disintegration of the intact microorganism or its toxic products by host cells, mainly by phagocytes; and (2) the immune response, whether it involves antibody-mediated or cell-mediated immunity, actually potentiates the effectiveness of phagocytic cells in ridding the host of the foreign invaders.

Classically, the immune response has been classified as follows. *Innate immunity* is a genetically endowed aspect of immunity. It is relatively constant for a species throughout the lifespan of the individual members of that species and cannot be transferred. For example, to the best of our knowledge, humans are never susceptible to infection by distemper virus yet canine hosts are. In contrast, humans are more susceptible to highly virulent infections by *S. aureus* than are most other animal host species. (The udders of cows may be infected with *S. aureus* by their human handlers.) Innate immunity undoubtedly includes factors inherent in the skin or outer surface structures, the phagocytic cells, secretions and immune responsiveness of a species.

Acquired immunities may be actively or passively acquired during either natural or artificial immunization processes. *Active, naturally acquired immunity* is that immunity which an individual develops to a specific infectious agent following exposure to and recovery from disease induced by that agent. *Active, artificially acquired immunity* is that which an individual develops following vaccination or immunization with either a living attenuated (lessened virulence) microorganism (e.g., vaccinia virus), a dead microorganism or a product of a microorganism (e.g., diphtheria and tetanus toxoids, detoxified toxins retaining the immunogenicity of the toxin). *Passive, naturally acquired immunity* is the immunity that an individual receives from its mother in utero (e.g., maternal IgG in the human fetus) or shortly after birth. For example, colostrum, the first mother's milk, is rich in antibodies (IgA). *Passive, artificially acquired immunity* is immunity received following injection of serum from an immune individual. In the past, equine and bovine sera from animals immunized with diphtheria or tetanus toxoids were used in passive immunization. Currently in use are human gamma globulin preparations (containing anti-tetanus toxin antibodies and horse anti-rabies virus antibodies). Passive immunization with sera or gamma globulin is short-lived (the half-life of immunoglobulins is longest for human IgG, 25 days, see Chapter 3) and is effective for approximately 6 weeks. Except in experimental situations and in attempts to restore immunodeficient individuals, immunologically competent lymphoid cells are not routinely administered to humans. The transfer of lymphoid cells is referred to as *adoptive transfer.* As is discussed in Chapter 7, successful restoration of immune capacity to clear the infecting agent in children with chronic mucocutaneous candidiasis has been achieved using dialyzable transfer factors prepared from lymphoid cells of immune humans.

SUGGESTED READINGS

Braun, W.: *Bacterial Genetics* (2nd ed.; Philadelphia: W. B. Saunders Co., 1965).

Burnet, M.: Trauma and Local Infection, in *Cellular Immunology* (Carlton: Melbourne University Press; London: Cambridge University Press, 1969).

Davis, B. D., Dulbecco, R., Eisen, H. N., Ginsberg, H. S., Wood, W. B., Jr., and McCarty, M.: *Microbiology* (2nd ed.; Hagerstown, Md.: Harper & Row, 1973).

Finegold, S. M., Rosenblatt, J. E., Sutter, V. L., and Attebery, H. R.: *Scope Monograph on Anaerobic Infections* (Kalamazoo, Mich.: The Upjohn Co., 1972).

Marples, M. J.: Life on the human skin, Sci. Am. 220:108, 1969.

2 / Antigens and Immunogens

BASIC DEFINITIONS

As classically used, the term *antigen* implies both functional and reactive capacities. Functionally, an *antigen* is any substance which when introduced into an organism induces an immune response. For many years humoral antibody production was the aspect of the immune response that received major attention. *Antibodies (immunoglobulins)* are reactive with the stimulating antigen in some detectable manner. It is now known that the immune response to a given antigen may also result in increased numbers of specifically reactive lymphocytes. There are two groups of specifically reactive lymphocytes. One group consists of memory cells for the production of antibody while the other group of cells is involved in cell-mediated immunity and lacks the capacity to produce humoral antibody. Both antibody and these specialized lymphocytes react with *the antigen used as the immunizing agent (immunogen)*. The *immunogenicity of an antigen* refers to its capacity to stimulate an immune response under a given set of conditions. Such conditions include factors characteristic of the individual being immunized such as species, genetic endowment, age and state of health as well as factors inherent in the immunogen such as its physical state, chemical composition and degree of complexity. The immunizing agent can be mixed with *substances which augment the immune response (adjuvants)*.

There are materials which in themselves are not immunogenic but when linked covalently to carrier molecules function as antigenic groups that direct the specificity of the immune response. Such materials are referred to as *haptens*. Haptenic substances will combine with antibody once it is formed.

WHAT KINDS OF SUBSTANCES ARE GOOD IMMUNOGENS?

Natural Biologic Substances

In general, the more "foreign" in chemical composition and structure the antigen is to the individual being immunized, the more

13

immunogenic that antigen is in that particular individual. Proteins are, for the most part, excellent immunogens as are certain large *complex polysaccharides,* e.g., the pneumococcal capsular polysaccharides and human blood group substances. Oligosaccharides are haptens, being nonimmunogenic themselves, but when covalently bonded to a high molecular weight substance stimulate an immune response. Certain homopolysaccharides such as cellulose or glycogen are not immunogenic, while others such as dextrans are. Lipids alone are not immunogenic but when bound to carrier molecules or physically adsorbed to proteins may function as haptens. Nucleic acids are also hapten antigens. Bacteriophage deoxyribonucleic acid (DNA), being markedly different in the composition of methylated bases from the DNA of mammalian cells, is immunogenic as are heat-denatured mammalian cell DNA preparations that have been salt-linked to methylated bovine serum albumin. Bacterial and mammalian cell ribosomes, containing both ribonucleic acid (RNA) and proteins, may be immunogenic. *Particulate antigens* such as viruses, bacteria and foreign erythrocytes are usually more potent immunogens than are soluble antigens. From the study of natural antigens it is apparent that most immunogens possess a molecular weight of 10,000 or greater. As in all of biology exceptions do exist, e.g., the polypeptide hormone glucagon with a molecular weight of 3,800 can be immunogenic as can insulin (molecular weight of 6,000) and several other hormones.

Artificial and Synthetic Immunogens

The chemical and structural features of an antigen which impart immunogenicity and specificity have been more readily elucidated through the study of artificial and synthetic antigens. Landsteiner was the first to study artificial antigens created by covalently linking organic radicals (haptens) through diazotization to the aromatic amino acids of a protein carrier. Such conjugated azoproteins are capable of stimulating antibodies reactive with the hapten alone, or reactive with the hapten coupled to a completely different carrier protein as well as antibodies reactive only with the carrier protein used in immunization. From these studies the following aspects of the relationship between chemical structure and immunogenicity were established. (1) The spatial arrangement of the acid radical is a significant factor in the specific immunogenicities and antigenic reactivities of the acid-coupled azoproteins. (2) The polar CONH-linkage enhances immunogenicity. (3) The length of an aliphatic chain coupled to a protein influences the specificity of the complex in that antibodies against short chains react specifically only with the homologous immunizing antigen. A difference of only one or two carbon atoms changes the specificity of the shorter chains. However, antisera prepared against longer aliphatic chains contain antibodies reactive with not only the homologous immunogen but also with similar antigens possessing lesser chain lengths. (4) Terminal amino acids appear to play a role in the immunogenic specificity of proteins. (5) Rather small structural alterations in the organic radical used as hapten dramatically affect the resultant immune response.

In more recent years, synthetic polypeptide antigens offer distinct advantages for studying more precisely the chemical and physical characteristics necessary for effective immunogenicity. With such antigens the size of the molecule can be controlled and the basic repeating units can be varied. The role of molecular conformation can be studied. The net charge of the molecule can also be controlled. From such studies the following facts have emerged. (1) Most homopolymers of amino acids are either not immunogenic or very poor immunogens. (2) D-amino acid polymers are immunogenic only in a low dose range. (3) Linear, random copolymers consisting of two different amino acids are more immunogenic than homopolymers. (4) Antibodies to naturally occurring L-peptides do not cross-react with D-peptides. (5) Linear, random copolymers consisting of three or four different L-amino acids are immunogenic in most species. (6) An optimal distance must exist between the immunogenic structure and the core or "backbone" of the molecule. The structure depicted in Figure 2-1 with a backbone of lysine residues and side chain "whiskers" consisting of DL-alanine linked to a terminal dipeptide of tyrosine-glutamine is a potent immunogen. By merely reversing the

Fig. 2-1.—Immunogenic and nonimmunogenic polypeptide structures containing identical amino acids. *L-lysine backbone* = polylysine; *DL-alanine* = poly-DL-alanine; and *tyrosine, glutamine* = poly (tyrosine, glutamic acid). (Redrawn from McDevitt, H. O., and Sela, M.: J. Exp. Med. 122:517, 1965.)

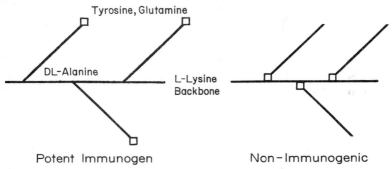

Potent Immunogen   Non-Immunogenic

position of the chemical "whiskers" in relation to the backbone portion of the molecule, a nonimmunogenic substance is created. The amino acid sequence of the primary structure influences the secondary structural folding of the molecule. Also, based on studies conducted with synthetic immunogens, the immune response has been shown to be under genetic control of the animal being immunized.

ANTIGENIC DETERMINANT, VALENCE
AND IMMUNODOMINANT GROUP

Those portions of an antigen molecule which induce an immune response and which, in turn, react with antibody or sensitized lymphocytes (i.e., impart specificity to the immune response) are referred to as *antigenic determinants*. The total number of antigenic determinants per antigen molecule is the *valence* of that antigen. Those determinants which are situated on the exterior of the antigen molecule are those whose function is readily measured, e.g., by binding with antibody. Structural alteration of the antigen molecule as in enzymatic degradation reveals inner determinants as well as, perhaps, altered determinants. The likelihood exists that some determinant structures may be destroyed by such degradation. The precise nature and number of antigenic determinants for practically all natural antigens is unknown. Of the natural antigens, serum albumins have been best characterized and contain six to seven antigenic determinants per molecule of undegraded albumin. For protein antigens the number of amino acids in an antigenic determinant is about five; for carbohydrate antigens such as dextran the optimal number of hexose units in the antigenic determinant is approximately six. For the nucleic acid hapten antigens an antigenic determinant consists of six to eight nucleotides.

An *immunodominant group* is that portion of the antigenic determinant which is crucial in conferring immunogenicity to the determinant and provides the greatest binding energy during its interaction with antibody. In some systems it is critical that the immunodominant group be situated in a terminal position in the molecule, while in others it seems unimportant whether the immunodominant group is buried or in a terminal position in the primary structure of the immunogen. Undoubtedly, immunodominant groups contribute considerably to or are actually exposed in a specified tertiary structure of the antigenic molecule.

The accessibility of antigenic determinants appears to be a major factor in the immunogenicity of a substance. Alterations of tertiary or quarternary structure of an antigen, as in enzymatic degradation, would bare "new" antigenic determinants. Yet not all degradative processes lead to a loss of tertiary structure of antigenic determinants. Using limited enzymatic cleavage, Sela and Arnon have described a 20-amino acid "loop" from the lysozyme molecule which is not only reactive with antibody to lysozyme but also is immunogenic when linked to a synthetic polypeptide carrier molecule. The resultant antibody reacts with both the 20-amino acid "loop" and intact lysozyme. Apparently, the immunodominant portions of the lysozyme molecule were retained in the conformation of the 20-amino acid "loop."

IMMUNIZATION AND THE IMMUNE RESPONSE

Genetic Capacity of the Individual Being Immunized

Later, more extensive descriptions of the lymphoid cell populations involved in the immune response are discussed. At this point in your learning it is sufficient to accept that the cells responsive to antigen in the formation of antibody immunoglobulins are called B lymphocytes or B cells, as depicted in Figure 2-2. Some B cells develop into immunoglobulin-secreting cells (plasma cells). In contrast, the cells responsible for mediating specific cellular immunity are called T lymphocytes or T cells. Upon initial contact with antigen these cells appear to increase in number and always remain identifiable as lymphocytes. For the induction of antibody responses to certain antigens a collaboration between T and B cells is necessary. Antigens inducing these responses as well as resultant antibody responses are called T cell-dependent or thymic-dependent antigens.

From studies with synthetic haptens and natural antigens in inbred strains of mice and guinea pigs, it is clear that a relationship exists between an animal's genetic endowment and its immune responsiveness. Those individuals which form antibodies to a given antigen are *responders* and those that do not are *nonresponders.* The gene(s) responsible for immune responsiveness to a given antigen appear to be linked, at least in mice, to the genes responsible for histocompatibility antigens. McDevitt and Benacerraf have identified several autosomal dominant genes, each of which is concerned with the capacity to form specific immune responses to a given antigen. Immune responsiveness is characterized by both sustained antibody formation and cell-mediated immunity. These genes appear to affect the recognition of antigen by the lymphoid cells of the animal's immune system and may be expressed only on T cells. Many natural antigens are fairly complex

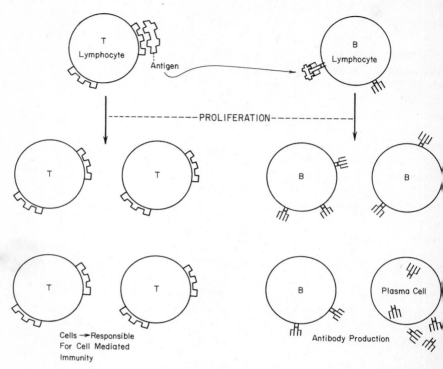

Fig. 2-2.—Schematic representation of antigen-induced proliferation of antigen-specific B and T lymphocytes.

immunogens possessing large numbers of diverse antigenic determinants. Thus, Sela has postulated that these strain-dependent variations in the immune response might go undetected because of the animal's ability to respond to a portion of the total number of determinants present in the immunogen.

Immunization versus Immunologic Unresponsiveness and Antigen Dose

For the purpose of stimulating an adequate immune response (e.g., high levels of antibody in the circulation) an optimal amount of antigen is required. This dose is referred to as an immunogenic dose. Amounts of antigen above or below this dose produce lesser, and in some instances, no immune response. This unresponsiveness is antigen-specific and further attempts to immunize such an individual with immunogenic doses of that particular antigen fail for prolonged periods of time. This state of specific unresponsiveness is termed *immunologic tolerance.* Adequate explanations do not exist for the induction of tolerance either with large quantities (high zone tolerance) or with minute quantities (low zone tolerance) of antigen.

The specific set of circumstances in which mice can be made refractory to antibody production in response to the injection of large doses of pneumococcal polysaccharide was originally described by Felton and termed immunologic paralysis. Since such animals can at some later date (e.g., 12 months later) respond in a detectable fashion to that antigen, it has been argued that these animals are not actually paralyzed from producing antibody but that antigen persisting in the tissues combines with the antibody being produced. Therefore, antibody is not detectable by routine serologic methods.

Even though definitive knowledge concerning the induction of tolerance does not exist, studies of the phenomenon have led to recent observations which aid in the selection of an adequate immunogenic dose of antigen for use in purposeful immunizations and also give insight as to why certain humans develop immune responses against self antigens. In mice, Weigle and associates found that both T and B cells could be rendered unresponsive to human gamma globulin (HGG) as antigen and suggested that certain T and B cells possess receptors for antigens contained in the HGG. Moreover, they showed that only one cell type need be made unresponsive for immunologic unresponsiveness to a given antigen to exist in the whole animal. Lesser amounts of antigen are needed to induce tolerance in T cells.

The tolerant state has been abrogated in inbred animals by the transfer of lymphoid cells from normal (not tolerant) individuals. Mitchison terminated low zone tolerance in mice following injection of antigen-treated thymus cells (T cells). In rabbits made tolerant at birth with bovine serum albumin (BSA, high zone tolerance), Weigle was able to terminate the tolerant state following immunization with antigens related to, but not identical to, the antigen used to induce tolerance (*tolerizing antigen*). He suggests that the tolerant rabbits, upon termination of unresponsiveness, made antibody against only those determinants shared between the tolerizing antigen and the related antigen. After several subsequent injections of the tolerizing antigen (BSA) the rabbits returned to the BSA-unresponsive state. Mitchison had evidence indicating that low zone tolerance is T cell tolerance while high zone tolerance represents tolerance of both B and T cell populations to the specific tolerizing antigen. Also, evidence exists to indicate that antibody formation may precede the establishment of tolerance to a given antigen.

Immune responsiveness to certain antigens such as flagellin (flagel-

lar protein of *Salmonella adelaide*) in rats appears to require cooperation between T and B cells. Parish chemically modified flagellin by
acetoacetylation and observed that as the extent of acetoacetylation
increased, the capacity to bind antibody to the native flagellin decreased. The acetoacetylated flagellin behaved as a tolerizing antigen
in the induction of antibody formation but as an excellent immunogen
for the induction of cell-mediated immunity. Parish has suggested that
the development of antibody production and cell-mediated immunity
to a given antigen are opposing processes. If so, the role of T cells
appears crucial in either process with this antigen. The altered state of
the flagellin in the acetoacetylated derivative undoubtedly created a
new set of antigenic determinants to which the rats were unresponsive
with respect to antibody production.

For the initiation of a readily detectable immune response, the
proper concentration and tertiary molecular structure of a given
antigen is necessary to interact with antigen-reactive members of T
and/or B cell populations.

CHEMICAL NATURE AND PHYSICAL STATE OF ANTIGEN
AND ANTIGEN PROCESSING

Based on the observation that virtually all antigens which stimulate
strong, sustained cell-mediated immune responses contain structural
lipid, Coon and Hunter synthesized lauryl BSA (bovine serum albumin [BSA] conjugated to lauric anhydride [dodecanoic acid]) and
examined its immunogenicity in comparison with that of BSA in
guinea pigs. When BSA was injected into the footpads of guinea pigs,
only antibody production was induced. But, when lauryl BSA was
similarly injected, cell-mediated immunity with little or no antibody
production was elicited. Using I^{125} labeled antigens they noted that
BSA localized in the follicles of the draining lymph node (sites where
B lymphocytes differentiate into antibody producing cells under the
influence of antigen), while lauryl BSA localized mainly in the
thymic-dependent areas of the node (paracortical and outer cortical
regions where T cells predominate). These results clearly indicate that
lipids enhance the production of cell-mediated immune responses by
promoting localization of certain antigens in areas of lymphoid tissue
rich in T cells.

The physical form of an antigen is of great significance in the
induction of an immune response. Proteins tend to aggregate in
solution and are usually excellent immunogens. Heat aggregation may
even improve the immunogenic potency of protein antigens. But,

when a solution of antigenic protein is centrifuged at 100,000 × g for several hours to sediment aggregates, the resultant solution (at comparable dosage levels to uncentrifuged protein solution) induces specific immunologic tolerance. Particulate antigens such as microorganisms, sheep erythrocytes and other mammalian cells are phagocytizable substances. Much effort has been put forth toward defining the role of phagocytic cells, especially macrophages, in the induction of the immune response.

The original work of Fishman and Adler implicated macrophages as cells which "processed" antigen producing ribonucleic acid (RNA) and/or RNA-antigen fragments as activated or "super" antigen which then influenced lymphocytes, in some manner, to produce antibody. This mechanism of antigen processing currently is controversial. Nevertheless, macrophages apparently are necessary for the immunogenesis by particulate antigens. A number of investigators have shown that macrophage-bound antigens (proteins, hapten-conjugated proteins and sheep erythrocytes) are capable of activating T cells. Activated T cells mediate cell-mediated immunity and also facilitate antibody production by B cells. Macrophage-bound antigen actually induces cell-mediated immunity but only primes the animals for the production of serum antibody, i.e., increases the number of antigen-reactive T cells which serve as "helper" cells for B cells. The macrophages need not be viable in order to exert these effects. Tuberculin (purified protein derivative, PPD) bound to macrophages induces only cell-mediated immunity to PPD while free soluble PPD stimulates only humoral antibody in guinea pigs.

Of the total amount of antigen injected only a very small portion is responsible for triggering the immune response. Macrophages may augment this process by removing excess antigen and preventing the establishment of high zone tolerance. Ehrenreich and Cohn have clearly shown that alveolar macrophages are capable of degrading protein antigens within the secondary lysosomes. Since only single amino acids and certain dipeptides are capable of diffusing out of the lysosome into the cytoplasm, it was concluded that such cells probably do not function in antigen processing. Dendritic cells (also called dendritic macrophages) present in organized lymphoid tissues are thought to trap and/or concentrate antigen in immunogenesis. The molecular conformation of antigen as presented to B and/or T cells in either the presence or absence of antibody may determine whether that cell undergoes an immune response or becomes tolerant. Obviously, a great deal of uncertainty still enshrouds the exact role of macrophages in the initiation and perpetuation of immune responses.

Retention of antigenic fragments in the tissues of a rabbit after immunization has been studied by Garvey and Campbell. Radio-labeled antigen was found in the parenchymal cells of the liver for a prolonged period (over 1 year). Garvey has suggested that continued antigenic stimulation necessary for maintaining the immune response is provided by the periodic release of antigen as individual parenchymal cells die.

ADJUVANTS

Certain substances (*adjuvants*) are capable of augmenting the immunogenicity of antigens. Such substances include aluminum salts (e.g. alum), sodium alginate, bacterial endotoxins, *Bordetella pertussis*, bacillus Calmette-Guérin (BCG) and other mycobacteria. Complete Freund's adjuvant consists of mineral oil containing dead tubercle bacilli (or other mycobacteria) and an emulsifying agent. The antigen in an aqueous medium is incorporated into the oil containing mycobacteria so that a water-in-oil emulsion results. Incomplete Freund's adjuvant does not contain the mycobacteria. Oligomers of nucleic acids and certain synthetic polynucleotides such as double-stranded polyadenylic:polyuridylic acid (poly AU) exert marked adjuvant effect when injected with antigen.

The effectiveness of adjuvants has been attributed to both retardation of antigen destruction, resulting in the maintenance of immunogenic doses of antigen in the tissues, and provocation of the inflammatory response. Complete Freund's adjuvant induces granuloma formation in animals. It has been suggested that within such granulomatous sites increased concentrations of hydrogen ions and proteolytic enzymes exist as a result of the host response to the mycobacteria in the adjuvant. In examining this possibility, Weigle and associates used the induction of thyroiditis as a model. Homologous rabbit thyroglobulin in complete Freund's adjuvant induces thyroiditis whereas the injection of aqueous solutions of thyroglobulin does not. But, when rabbits were injected with aqueous preparations of homologous thyroglobulin partially degraded in vitro with pepsin at acid pH, they produced antibody reactive with the native (untreated) thyroglobulin and developed thyroiditis.

Braun has offered a mechanism of action for all substances which exert an adjuvant action based on the observation that such substances cause, to some degree, cell necrosis and liberation of oligmers of host cell nucleic acids. In the presence of antigen or substances which alter permeability of lymphocyte membranes, oligonucleotides have been shown to stimulate the rate of increase in numbers of antibody-forming cells. This mode of action involves cyclic adenosine 3′, 5′-monophosphate (cAMP) of the lymphocyte. Synthetic polynucleotides, especially poly AU, enhance both antibody and cell-mediated immune responses to antigens. An elevation in cAMP in cells involved in the immune response enhances the activity of these cells. If antigen and poly AU are injected simultaneously with a stabilizer of cAMP (e.g., theophylline), the adjuvant effect of poly AU is enhanced either in vivo or in vitro.

The efficacy of some adjuvants may be the result of activation of T cells by antigens inherent in the adjuvants. Consequently, soluble factors are released by the T lymphocytes (some of which may be Braun's nucleic acid oligmers) which, in turn, activate macrophages and/or B lymphocytes. Maillard and Bloom have shown that both pertussis vaccine and mycobacterial adjuvants appear to activate T cells in this manner. Both materials augment a primary antibody response to antigen (sheep erythrocytes) by mouse spleen cells.

ROUTE OF INJECTION

The site into which antigen is introduced into an organism influences the immune response. Most antigen administered intravenously is entrapped in the spleen in a relatively short time. For example, when bovine gamma globulin (BGG) is injected into the jugular vein of guinea pigs antibody is subsequently produced. When the same antigen is injected into the mesenteric vein of guinea pigs tolerance is induced. It is possible that the antigen is deaggregated in the liver or disposed of there by Kupffer cells and that either the monomeric form or the amount (low zone tolerance) reaching the immunocompetent cells in the spleen induces tolerance. It has been known for many years that certain hapten antigens such as picryl chloride when injected into the skin bind to body proteins and then are capable of inducing both antibody and cell-mediated immunity to the hapten. If, however, guinea pigs are first fed picryl chloride and then injected intradermally with the hapten, neither antibody nor cell-mediated immunity is produced.

Unless adjuvants are used in the injection mixture, antigen is not retained at the injection site but is disseminated throughout the body via the vascular and lymphatic circulations. Since the lymphatics drain much of the body surface areas, substances injected subcutaneously are carried by lymph vessels into lymph nodes as well as into the circulation.

Soluble antigens such as proteins seem to persist in the extracellula spaces of the body while particulate antigens such as bacteria are readily phagocytized. Nossal and Ada have cited the rapid clearance by phagoyctes of polypeptides composed of D-amino acids and many high molecular weight substances. Rats injected intravenously with a labeled soluble antigen (radiolabeled flagellin) retained only 1–2% of the label in their sera and 0.07% in their spleens 12 hours later.

When intradermal and subcutaneous routes are employed, highes concentrations of antigen are localized in the lymph nodes draining the area of the injection site. The induction of delayed hypersensitivity (cell-mediated immunity) is favored by introduction of antigen by dermal routes. Antigen has been shown to localize on the extensive surface areas of dendritic macrophages where it is available for interaction with lymphoid cells. One opinion is that it is at this site (dendritic cell + antigen + T and/or B lymphocytes) that the immune response is initiated in the spleen and other peripheral lymphoid tissues.

Immune deviation (also known as split or partial tolerance) is a phenomenon shown to exist for certain antigens and involves intravenous injection of antigen shortly (usually 24 hours but can be as long as 2–3 days) before injection of antigen in complete Freund's adjuvant. The immune response which ensues is mainly an antibody response. In fact, this procedure has been used to prevent specifically the formation of cell-mediated immunity in several experimental situations.

A competition occurs in which an immune response is made against only one of two strong antigenic determinants when one is injected simultaneously with or within several days of the other. This phenomenon is called *antigenic competition*. The mechanism of antigenic competition is not well understood but may involve competition for the "helper" effect of T cells in collaboration with B cell responses. However, the method of immunization is important and this phenomenon appears to be dose-dependent.

ANTIGENS AND THE IMMUNE RESPONSE

The immune response serves as an adaptive response of the living organism to antigenic stimuli of both exogenous and endogenous origin. Among external antigens encountered naturally are microorganisms and pollens. In blood transfusions and tissue transplantation *alloantigens* (genetically inherited antigens which are present within a species but not in all members of that species; formerly called isoantigens) may be introduced into an individual from an external source. Individuals carrying a given alloantigen do not usually respond immunologically to that antigen. Included in the category of internal antigens that may arise within an individual are the variety of substances known to be self or autoantigens and tumor-specific transplantation antigens (TSTA's).

The existence of *heterogenetic antigens,* at times, confuses the issue of whether an antigenic stimulus has been exogenous or endogenous. An antigen is termed heterogenetic when it is found in a variety of phylogenetically unrelated species. Forssman antigens are found in many animals (in the tissues of guinea pigs, cats, horses and chickens) and in some bacterial species. These antigens are defined by their capacity to induce in rabbits (a species which lacks Forssman antigen) hemolytic antibodies for sheep erythrocytes. Some humans with infectious mononucleosis develop *heterophil antibodies* which agglutinate sheep erythrocytes and this fact is used diagnostically. The precise immunogen stimulating this response is not defined. Heterophil antibodies also develop in humans with serum sickness. To distinguish among such heterophil antibodies (antibodies reactive with heterogenetic antigens) absorption tests are employed. Antibodies of infectious mononucleosis are absorbed by bovine erythrocytes but not by guinea pig kidney; heterophil antibodies in the sera of patients with serum sickness are absorbable by both bovine erythrocytes and guinea pig kidney. Other heterogenetic antigens used diagnostically involve bacteria. Antibodies formed during the course of rickettsial infections in humans react with the polysaccharide O antigens of Proteus OX strains (this reaction is called the Weil-Felix reaction). In humans infected with *M. pneumoniae,* serum antibodies are present which will agglutinate streptococcus MG. Certain streptococci (group A, beta hemolytic streptococci) contain antigens in their cell walls and cytoplasmic membranes which are similar, if not identical, to components of human and rabbit hearts. Moreover, certain of the group A, beta hemolytic streptococci share antigens in common with the basement membrane of the human glomerulus. Such streptococci are called nephritogenic. Some enteric bacilli contain an antigen (Kunin) in common with the human intestinal mucosa. The rabbit, guinea pig, rat and mouse all share tissue antigens (histocompatability antigens) with *S. aureus, S. albus* and *S. pyogenes.*

EXOGENOUS MICROBIAL ANTIGENS

Much of our knowledge concerning microbial antigens has been gained from the study of bacterial antigens and, more recently, of viral antigens. The outermost portion of the bacterial cell consists of a slime layer and, in some instances, a capsule. In the pneumococci the polysaccharide capsule is antigenic and protects the pneumococcus from phagocytosis. In the presence of antibody which binds to the capsule and causes it to swell and become "sticky," the pneumococci are readily ingested by phagocytic cells. The bacterial cell wall contains a mosaic of complex chemical structures foreign to the animal host. With specific reference to the salmonellae (Fig. 2-3), the outermost antigen which forms when the bacteria are growing in host tissues is referred to as K antigen and, in certain species, is designated as Vi antigen. When Vi antigen is present it appears to be composed of carbohydrate material. In flagellated species the flagellar antigens are designated as H antigens. The O antigen complex (endotoxin) of the gram-negative enteric bacilli is situated in the membrane-cell wall complex of these bacteria. Antibodies to these structures usually react with the O side chain carbohydrate determinants of the complex. These carbohydrate moieties and, in turn, the antigenic specificity of the O antigen may be altered in the salmonellae by a process known as phage conversion. Under the influence of the genetic material (DNA) of certain bacteriophage the carbohydrate structure is antigenically altered. Even a change in linkage results in conformational changes which are immunologically recognized. For years the nucleoprotein components of bacteria have been recognized as antigenic. The soluble bacterial exotoxins which are either membrane-bound or secreted into the growth medium have been considered for many years as classic examples of highly immunogenic protein antigens. More recent information indicates that some bacterial exotoxins are not only proteins but complexes of proteins and lipids or proteins and carbohydrates.

Through the utilization of the tools of molecular biology and electronmicroscopy the structure of viruses has been elucidated. Viruses are basically composed of nucleic acid and protein, although

Fig. 2-3.—Representation of external antigens of gram-negative bacilli.

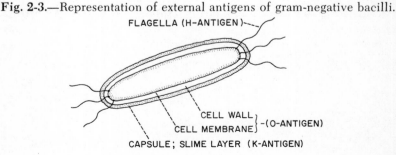

FLAGELLA (H-ANTIGEN)

CELL WALL
CELL MEMBRANE } -(O-ANTIGEN)

CAPSULE; SLIME LAYER (K-ANTIGEN)

some viruses are structurally complex and also contain carbohydrate and lipid moieties. The intact structures of the virus exterior are excellent antigens and are mainly protein or, in some instances, lipoproteins and/or glycoproteins.

The antigenic structure of fungal parasites is not as well known as that of bacteria and viruses. Certain fungi such as *Cryptococcus neoformans* exist naturally as soil saprophytes with little capsular material. However, upon infection of the animal host a capsule appears which is different chemically from that produced by this fungus in the soil and which protects it from phagocytic destruction. This is but one problem which exists in attempts to define antigenic structures of fungi. Similarly, members of the bacterial genus Borrelia (causative agents of relapsing fever) change their surface antigenic structure in the infected human for as many as five or more "relapses." No sooner does the host respond immunologically to the surface antigens of one phase of this bacterium than the parasite disappears only to re-emerge with a new array of surface antigens. Protozoan parasites which live in several animal hosts during their complex sexual and asexual life cycles also undergo morphologic alterations within a given host. Many of these growth phases occur within host cells, thereby protecting the parasite from the host's immune response. Thus, a definition of protozoan antigens is an awesome task as is a comprehension of a meaningful immune response to these parasites.

ENDOGENOUS ANTIGENS

Alloantigens*

The blood group (erythrocyte) antigens as well as transplantation antigens, several soluble proteins (haptoglobins, transferrins and certain beta-lipoproteins) and some antigens in immunoglobulin molecules are alloantigenic (formerly called isoantigenic) within the human species. The existence of such molecular differences within a species is indicative of the genetic individuality of each member. In the human, transfusion reactions have occurred most commonly against the erythrocyte antigens but may result from immunization to any of the other alloantigens.

BLOOD GROUP SUBSTANCES.—There are many blood group antigen systems. Among those most commonly identified in clinical immu-

*Alloantigens (allotypic antigens): intraspecies antigens; present in some, but not all, members of a species. Isoantigens (isotypic antigens): species-specific antigens; present in all members of a species. Idiotypic antigens: individually specific antigens as in the Fab regions of an immunoglobulin molecule (see Chapter 3).

nology and blood banking procedures are the ABO, MN, Ss, P, Rh, Lutheran, Kell, Kidd, Lewis, and Duffy antigens. Only the ABO and Rh antigen systems are briefly included in this text.

ABO antigens.—The ABO system is unique in that it is the only alloantigen system in which naturally occurring antibodies (agglutinins) regularly exist. These antigens are mucopeptides ranging in molecular weight from 200,000 to 1,000,000. The active antigenic determinant is carbohydrate in nature.

Persons possessing O gene (blood group O) display H antigen specificity on their erythrocytes. Individuals of blood group A possess A gene and A antigen on their red blood cells. Similarly, group B individuals exhibit B antigen on their erythrocytes and AB individuals display both A and B antigens on their erythrocytes. This system consists of three allelic genes (A, B and O). Two alleles exist in each individual with A and B genes being dominant over O. For example, an individual of blood group A may be homozygous (AA) or heterozygous (AO) genetically. The offspring of a couple whose genotypes are AO and BO may be: AB genetically and phenotypically; OO genetically and O phenotypically; AO genetically and A phenotypically; and BO genetically and B phenotypically. Actually minor variations exist in the antigenicity of both blood groups A and B. The variations in group A are well established. Among the humans of blood group A, 80% are A_1; A_2 and A_3 antigens as well as other variations in A antigen do exist.† The variations in the B antigen are not yet clearly defined.

The O antigen (H substance) is a truly heterogenetic antigen being present not only in man but in a variety of other species. Evidence exists to suggest that the H gene is independent of the ABO alleles. H substance appears to serve as a precursor upon which the enzymes expressed by either the A or B genes act. Consequently, in group O individuals the H substance is not altered and thereby is not only fully expressed but also exposed on the surface of the erythrocyte. This may be more fully appreciated by examining the carbohydrate structure of the nonreducing ends of the chains of the antigenic molecules. Those of blood group O contain as the active H substance:

β-D-galactose-(1 → 3 or 1 → 4)-N-acetyl-D-glucosamine
2 ↑

1 |
α-L-fucose

---

†A_1 cells possess 4 to 5 times the number of A-reactive sites as do A_2 cells. A_2 cells possess more H-active sites than do A_1 cells.

In the blood group A substance, a residue of α-N-acetyl galactosamine is attached to the β-D-galactose of the above structure. In B substance a residue of α-galactose is linked to the β-D-galactose of the H substance.

A, B and H substances are found on cells of the body other than erythrocytes and in 75% of all humans (known as secretors) in body secretions such as saliva, sweat, gastric mucin, meconium, pancreatic secretions and ovarian cyst fluid.

Naturally Occurring Antibodies to Blood Group Antigens.—Even though antibody immunoglobulins are presented in the next chapter, a brief description of the naturally occurring antibodies directed against A and B substances is included here. Individuals of blood group O contain both anti-A and anti-B antibodies in their sera. These agglutinins are of the IgM and IgG classes. Individuals of blood group A contain only anti-B antibody which is of the IgM class predominantly, while group B individuals contain anti-A activity in their sera which is also predominantly IgM. Upon receipt of antigenic stimulation (e.g., an incompatible transfusion) an individual will form mainly IgG class antibodies to these antigens. The existence of these naturally occurring agglutinins has never been adequately explained. However, the most likely and widely accepted explanation is as follows. Since A- and B-like carbohydrate substances are widely distributed phylogenetically, the human receives antigenic stimuli via the gastrointestinal tract through plant products and bacteria which contain the A- and B-like carbohydrates. Because of the existence of immunologic tolerance to self antigens, the immune system of an individual will only recognize as "foreign" those antigenic structures which that person lacks. Thus, an individual of blood group A will not be immunized by heterogenetic polysaccharides containing A-like substance but will react to B substance, forming anti-B antibodies. This concept explains the existence of anti-A and anti-B in the sera of blood group O individuals and their absence in the sera of blood group AB individuals.

Rh Antigens.—The Rh antigens comprise a complex blood group antigen system of great clinical importance because of the fact that maternal immunization to an Rh antigen (D, Rh_o) present in the fetus and absent in the mother may result in erythroblastosis fetalis (hemolytic disease of the newborn). This antigen system is involved in a more severe erythroblastosis fetalis although incompatibilities in ABO, Duffy or Kell systems are occasionally responsible. In instances in which antibodies of anti-A or anti-B reactivity may pass through the placenta into a fetus containing the A or B blood group substance, fetal tissues possessing A or B substance will absorb the antibody and consequently the fetal erythrocytes are spared from extensive hemolysis. Erythroblastosis fetalis occurs more frequently in newborns of Rh-negative (lacking D, Rh_0 antigen) mothers and Rh-positive fathers and more frequently in babies whose mothers have experienced multiple pregnancies. The disease occurs less in infants of Rh incompatible parents who are also ABO incompatible. In these circumstances the presumption is that as a result of the ABO incompatibility, maternal antibodies against the major blood group antigens rapidly remove fetal cells from the maternal circulation and thereby decrease the opportunity for the mother's immune system to be stimulated by the Rh antigen of the fetal erythrocytes.

The Rh antigens have never been precisely defined chemically, although evidence indicates that they may reside in membrane lipoproteins. Two schemes are used to identify these antigens. Wiener's nomenclature is probably more accurate in the definition of antigens and antigenic variations as they exist on the human red cells. He considers all genes which specify the Rh antigens as allelic and that each allele dictates a single large antigenic structure which consists of smaller antigenic determinants. On the other hand, the Fisher-Race scheme of nomenclature is more readily envisioned. Fisher considers the Rh locus to consist of three allelic pairs of closely linked genes, Cc, Dd, and Ee.

HISTOCOMPATIBILITY ANTIGENS.—The genetics of histocompatibility antigens is complex. Histocompatibility genes are located on chromosome regions designated as histocompatibility loci which determine the transplantation antigens on the surface of tissue cells. At each such locus a series of alleles may occur. In the human species two major histocompatibility systems have been described; namely, the ABO blood group antigens and the HL-A (human histocompatibility locus A) system. HL-A antigens exist on the surface of cells of human tissues and may serve as antigenic stimuli following transfusion since they are present on lymphocytes, reticulocytes, platelets and granulocytes.

At present, the exact number of HL-A antigens is not known. The HL-A factors have been separated on the basis of genetic studies into two segregant series (the LA or "first" and Four or "second" series). The chemical nature of these antigens is thought to be primarily protein or protein conjugated to polysaccharides, although the carbohydrate does not appear to be of significance in the immunogenicity of these molecules.

From each parent an individual receives one gene from each series and thereby the cells of each individual display four HL-A antigens (two of the LA series and two of the Four series which is the same as two haplotypes). These antigens are produced by closely linked genes. An LA and a Four antigen from one parent equals a haplotype. HL-A antigens are associated in haplotypes, one haplotype from each parent.

Over 95% of the possible alleles in both series can be recognized by serologic methods. The LA locus may specify more than 10 allelomorphic antigens while the Four locus may specify more than 20 different antigens. In each HL-A specificity the protein antigen may actually be very heterogenous and each established specificity may eventually be split into subgroups by new typing antisera with restricted specificities. For example, individuals displaying antigenic specificity for HL-A 1 may in reality not contain identical protein structures on their cells but only similar (and cross-reacting) structures.

The following terminology has been or is used in reference to tissue grafts. A skin graft from one site on the body to another site on the same individual is an *autograft.* A graft from one identical twin to the other (or from genetically identical or near identical individuals) is a *syngeneic graft* or *syngraft* (formerly isograft). A tissue graft from a genetically dissimilar member of the same species to another individual is designated as an *allograft* (formerly homograft). A tissue graft between dissimilar species had been referred to as an heterograft but is now designated as a *xenograft.*

For the successful transplantation of tissues from one human to another, the antigens of the donor and recipient tissues should be closely matched antigenically and be as nearly identical as possible. Otherwise, the grafted tissue is rejected by the immune system (cell-mediated immunity) of the recipient. In the recipient whose immune system is deficient or depressed, "foreign" (mismatched) donor lymphoid cells in the graft may respond immunologically to the recipient's tissue antigens. This situation is termed a *graft-versus-host (GVH)* reaction and may lead to death of the recipient.

Certain tissues may be transplanted successfully even though donor and recipient are histoincompatible. Cartilage is one such tissue. Because of the unique physicochemical nature of the substance secreted by the chondrocytes, the question arises as to whether immunization even occurs in the recipient. Billingham and Silvers cite experimental evidence that cartilage is not completely rejected in recipients who have been previously immunized with cartilage as antigen. Apparently, even in the face of immunization the "immune" lymphocytes are not able to reach and kill all viable chondrocytes surrounded by their secreted matrix.

Tumors which arise within an individual (autochthonous) may not

be destroyed for the same reason. Certain tumor types secrete si-
alomucins which may mask tumor-specific transplantation antigens
(TSTA's). Also, since some tumor antigens are identical to human
embryonic antigens, the phenomenon of immunologic tolerance may
prevent the stimulation of an immune response effective in the killing
of the malignant cells.

Billingham and Silvers have separated allografts into two categories.
The *homovital grafts* are those in which the original transplanted cell
populations must retain viability. Examples are: skin, heart, kidneys
and lymphohematopoietic tissues. It is in this category that donor and
recipient antigens should be closely matched. *Homostatic grafts* are
those which are necessary for mainly mechanical purposes. Examples
are: teeth, bone, fascia, cartilage, tendons and segments of blood
vessels. Viability, even at the time of transplantation, is not a necessity
since these grafts retain their physical properties adequately to fulfill
their physiologic functions.

Corneal transplants are successful as long as the corneal graft
remains avascular. In time, the donor stromal cells of the transplanted
cornea are replaced by recipient host cells and the cornea is no longer
vulnerable to immunologic rejection.

In studying the so-called immunologically privileged sites of the
body such as the brain, Medawar found that skin implanted into
animal brain did not evoke a graft rejection. This is explained by the
fact that lymphatic drainage is absent in the brain; thus immunization
does not occur. However, in animals previously sensitized by another
injection route with skin as antigen, rejection of skin grafted into the
brain was complete within 10 days. This latter observation is explained
by the fact that lymphocytes are able to enter virtually every tissue of
the body.

AUTOANTIGENS.—In the normally immunocompetent host, autoimmunization leading to disease apparently does not occur. Ehrlich's
thesis of "Horror Autotoxicus" implied that autoimmunization to self
antigens was incompatible with normal life. Individuals who are
victims of certain autoimmune diseases would undoubtedly agree. In
such persons immunologic tolerance to self antigens has seemingly
been abrogated. The possible mechanisms of induction are discussed
later in this text. In the human species autoantibodies and/or reactive
lymphocytes have been evoked to a variety of self antigens. Some of
these are: denatured H chains of IgG; DNA; RNA; histone; nucleoprotein; brain; peripheral nerve; erythrocyte antigens (those of the Rh
system in particular); heart; glomerular basement membrane; intes-

tinal mucosa; thyroglobulin; thyroid colloid; parietal cells; intrinsic factor; mitochondria; myoneural elements; sperm; and salivary duct cells.

TUMOR ANTIGENS.—Certain tumor antigens are specified by oncogenic viruses either directly or indirectly. Other tumor antigens are unique to each tumor and are not considered to be the products of viral genes. Another type of tumor antigen is a fetal antigen which is displayed on normal cells during the early development of the individual.

Malignant alterations of normal cells may be effected by physical agents (such as ionizing radiations), chemical carcinogens (e.g., coal tar derivatives) and by viruses in animal models. Both DNA and RNA viruses may be oncogenic in lower animals. For example, in mice, polyoma and SV40 viruses are DNA viruses which produce tumors, while the murine leukemia agents are RNA-containing viruses. A number of surface properties different from those of normal cells occur in the malignant transformation of a cell. Membrane antigens may be altered in such a way that the fully malignant cell displays different antigens from those of its normal counterpart (Fig. 2-4). These antigens are called tumor-specific transplantation antigens (TSTA's) and exist on the tumor cell membrane.

Currently, many investigators are attempting to utilize this difference in efforts to effect tumor rejection following immunization against TSTA's. At this time, four antigen systems have been identified with human cancers but have not really been proven to be TSTA's. (1) Epstein-Barr (EB) virus-related antigens are present on cultured lymphoblastoid cells. Antibodies to these antigens are present in patients with Burkitt's lymphoma, nasopharyngeal carcinoma, infectious mononucleosis and sarcoidosis. (2) S (sarcoma) antigens are present in cell lines derived from human sarcoma. Antibodies to these antigens are widespread among members of the human species but are present in highest titer in sarcoma patients, their near relatives and close contacts. (3) Two classes of malignant melanoma cell antigens and antibodies to them have been described. One is an intracellular antigen shared by all malignant melanomas and antibody to this antigen is present in highest titer in the sera of patients with malignant melanoma. The other antigen is a cell surface antigen distinct for each tumor and reactive antibody is present only in the patient from whom the tumor cells were derived. This second antigen is more likely a TSTA. (4) Fetal antigens have been identified which were exposed during fetal life and reactivated (or their genetic expression dere-

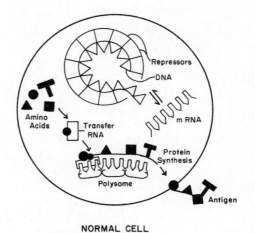

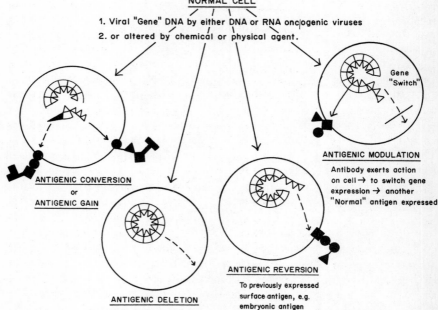

Fig. 2-4.—Possible ways in which normal cell surface antigens may be transformed.

pressed) during the malignant process. Several of these systems exist. Alpha$_1$-fetoprotein is present in the serum of patients with embryonal adenocarcinoma and hepatoma. The carcinoembryonic antigen (CEA) associated with carcinomas of the digestive tract should be an aid in the early diagnosis of intestinal malignancies, particularly carcinoma of the colon. A third fetal antigen, gamma-fetoprotein, has been described. This latter antigen exists in a proportion of all histologic types of tumors examined and is also present in certain benign as well as malignant tumors.

The Hellströms and their associates have demonstrated antigenic cross-reactivity between tumors of the same histologic type for seven human neoplasms (malignant melanomas, carcinomas of the colon, breast, testis, endometrium and ovary, and various sarcomas). These tumor-specific antigens are TSTA's since lymphocytes from 88–89% of patients bearing the same tumor type were cytotoxic for the cultured tumor cells.

SUGGESTED READINGS

Benacerraf, B., and McDevitt, H. O.: Histocompatibility-linked immune response genes, Science 175:273, 1972.

Billingham, R., and Silvers, W.: *The Immunobiology of Transplantation,* Foundations of Immunology Series, (Englewood Cliffs, N. J.: Prentice-Hall, Inc., 1971).

Borek, F. (ed.): *Immunogenicity,* Frontiers of Biology, Vol. 25 (Amsterdam-London: North Holland Pub. Co.; New York: American Elsevier Pub. Co., 1972).

Braun, W., Nakano, M., Jaraskova, L., Yajima, Y., and Jimenez, L.: Stimulation of Antibody-Forming Cells by Oligonucleotides of Known Composition, in Plescia, O. J., and Braun, W. (eds.): *Nucleic Acids in Immunology* (New York: Springer-Verlag, Inc., 1968).

Braun, W., Ishizuka, M., Yajima, Y., Webb, D., and Winchurch, R.: Spectrum and Mode of Action of Poly A:U in the Stimulation of Immune Responses, in Burs, R. F., and Braun, W. (eds.): *Biological Effects of Polynucleotides* (New York: Springer-Verlag, Inc., 1971).

Coon, J., and Hunter, R.: Selective induction of delayed hypersensitivity by a lipid conjugated protein antigen which is localized in thymus dependent lymphoid tissue, J. Immunol. 110:183, 1973.

Ehrenreich, B. A., and Cohn, Z. A.: Pinocytosis by macrophages, J. Reticuloendothel. Soc. 5:230, 1968.

Fishman, M., and Adler, F. L.: The role of macrophage RNA in the immune response, Cold Spring Harbor Symp. 32:343, 1967.

Garvey, J. S., and Campbell, D. H.: The retention of ^{35}S-labelled bovine serum albumin in normal and immunized rabbit liver tissue, J. Exp. Med. 105:361, 1957.

Garvey, J. S.: On the Role of Antigen Fragments and RNA in the Immune Response of Rabbits to a Soluble Antigen, in Plescia, O. J., and Braun, W. (eds.): *Nucleic Acids in Immunology* (New York: Springer-Verlag, Inc., 1968).

Gottlieb, A. A., and Schwartz, R. H.: Review: Antigen-RNA interactions, Cell. Immunol. 5:341, 1972.

Gottlieb, A. A., and Waldman, S. R.: The multiple functions of macrophages in immunity, CRC Critical Rev. Microbiol., Feb.:321, 1972.

Hellström, I., et al.: Demonstration of cell-mediated immunity to human neoplasms of various histological types, Int. J. Cancer 7:1, 1971.

Katz, D. H., and Benacerraf, B.: The regulatory influence of activated T cells on B cell responses to antigen, Adv. Immunol. 15:1, 1972.

Landsteiner, K.: The Specificity of Serological Reactions, Rev. ed. (Cambridge: Harvard University Press, 1945).

Maillard, J., and Bloom, B. R.: Immunological adjuvants and the mechanism of cell cooperation, J. Exp. Med. 136:185, 1972.

McDevitt, H. O., and Benacerraf, B.: Genetic control of specific immune responses, Adv. Immunol. 11:31, 1969.

McDevitt, H. O., and Landy, M. (eds.): Genetic Control of Immune Responsiveness (New York and London; Academic Press, 1972).

McDevitt, H. O., and Sela, M.: Genetic control of the antibody responses. I. Demonstration of determinant-specific differences in response to synthetic polypeptide antigens in two strains of inbred mice, J. Exp. Med. 122:517, 1965.

Mitchison, N. A.: Immunocompetent Cell Populations, in Landy, M., and Braun, W. (eds.): Immunological Tolerance (New York and London: Academic Press, 1969).

Möller, G.: Immunocyte triggering, Cell Immunol. 1:573, 1970.

Nossal, G. J. V., and Ada, G. L.: Antigens, Lymphoid Cells and the Immune Response (New York and London: Academic Press, 1971).

Parish, C. R.: Suppression of antibody formation and concomitant enhancement of cell-mediated immunity by acetoacetylated derivatives of Salmonella flagellin, Ann. N. Y. Acad. Sci. 181:108, 1971.

Sela, M.: Antigenicity: Some molecular aspects, Science 166:1365, 1969.

Sela, M.: Antigen Design and Immune Response, in The Harvey Lectures, Series 67 (New York and London: Academic Press, 1973).

Unanue, E. R.: The regulatory role of macrophages in antigenic stimulation, Adv. Immunol. 15:95, 1972.

Weigle, W. O.: Immunological unresponsiveness, Adv. Immunol. 16:61, 1973.

3 / Immunoglobulins

IMMUNOGLOBULINS

All antibody molecules are globulins but not all serum globulins are antibodies. By electrophoretic separation of serum proteins, antibody globulins are localized in the gamma globulin and occasionally beta globulin regions as diagrammed in Figure 3-1. The antibody portions of the serum globulins are referred to as *immunoglobulins.*

STRUCTURE AND PROPERTIES OF IMMUNOGLOBULINS

Each monomeric unit of immunoglobulin is composed of four polypeptide chains as shown in Figure 3-2. The two heavy (H) chains, each with a molecular weight of approximately 55,000, are held together with as many as five disulfide bonds. The H chains are class-specific, containing unique amino acid sequences which specify

Fig. 3-1.—Schematic representation of electrophoretic migration of serum proteins.

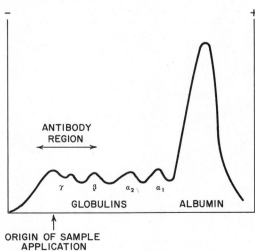

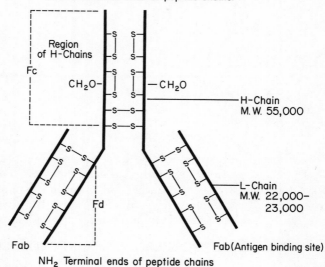

Fig. 3-2.—Basic structure of immunoglobulin molecule.

Fig. 3-3.—Basic structure of an IgG$_1$ molecule showing variable and constant regions (From Edelman, 1970 and 1971). L chain = 214 amino acids; H chain = 446 amino acids; V_L = variable region of light chain, amino acids 1–108; C_L = constant region of light chain, amino acids 109–214; V_H = variable region of heavy chain, amino acids 1–114; C_H1 = constant region of heavy chain, amino acids 119–220; C_H2 = constant region of heavy chain, amino acids 234–341; C_H3 = constant region of heavy chain, amino acids 342–446; CH_2O = carbohydrate; NH_2 = amino (N) terminus; PCA = pyrollidone carboxylic acid at N-terminus of H chain; $COOH$ = carboxy (C) terminus; Hinge region is area between C_H1 and C_H2.

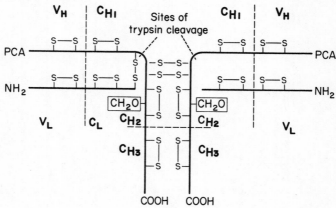

TABLE 3-1.—CHARACTERISTICS OF HUMAN IMMUNOGLOBULINS

PROPERTY	IMMUNOGLOBULIN CLASS				
	IgM	IgG	IgA	IgD	IgE
Molecular weight	890,000–1,000,000	150,000–160,000	Monomer: 170,000 Secretory: 390,000	150,000–~190,000	196,000–200,000
Sedimentation constant (S_{20w})	19S (24 and 32S polymers)	6.6–7S	Serum: 7, 11, and 15S	7S	7.8–8.2S
Carbohydrate content (%)	11.8	2–3	7.5–10	14.8	10.7
Valence	10	2	2/monomer	2	2
Subclasses	possibly 2	4 (IgG_1, IgG_2, IgG_3, and IgG_4)	2 (IgA_1 and IgA_2)		
H Chain	Mu	Gamma	Alpha	Delta	Epsilon
H chain allotypes		Gm (1–25) on $\gamma_{1,2,3}$ chains	Am on α 2 chains		
L chains*	$\frac{2}{3}$ κ $\frac{1}{3}$ λ	$\frac{2}{3}$ κ $\frac{1}{3}$ λ	$\frac{2}{3}$ κ $\frac{1}{3}$ λ	$\frac{2}{3}$ κ $\frac{1}{3}$ λ	$\frac{2}{3}$ κ $\frac{1}{3}$ λ
L chain allotypes			κ InV (1–3) in all classes		
Isotypes			λ (Oz) in all classes		

*Although inadequate amounts of human IgD and IgE are available, except for myeloma proteins, 2/3 of all Ig molecules are considered to contain kappa light chains.

39

their type; e.g., gamma (γ) heavy chains are found in the immunoglobulin G class (IgG). The disulfide bridges are usually concentrated near the center of the H chains and this area is usually rich in proline residues. This region of the immunoglobulin molecule is referred to as the *hinge* region (Fig. 3-3). The hinge region appears to impart rigidity to the molecule in this area, allowing the remainder of the molecule to be flexible. Confirmation of this flexibility is supported by the electronmicroscopic studies of the IgG molecule bound to antigen. The antigen appears to bind at the tips of the arms of the Y-shaped immunoglobulin. In the human species five classes of H chains exist: gamma (γ) chains in IgG; mu (μ) chains in IgM; alpha (α) chains in IgA; delta (δ) chains in IgD; and epsilon (ϵ) chains in IgE. Characteristics of human immunoglobulins are contained in Table 3-1. The two light (L) chains, each with a molecular weight of approximately 22,000 to 23,000, are of either the kappa (κ) or lambda (λ) type and are united with the two H chains. An H-L chain bridge is formed between the carboxy terminal amino acid (carboxy terminus) of the kappa light chain and an amino acid near the center of the human H chain (in IgG_1) and to amino acids nearer the amino terminus of the H chain in other classes and subclasses of immunoglobulins. In some IgA molecules, $IgA_2(Am_1+)$, absence of such H-L chain disulfide bonds has been described; the H and L chains in these molecules appear to be held together by noncovalent bonds. The lambda light chain appears linked to the H chain through the amino acid residue adjacent to the carboxy terminus of the L chain. These disulfide bridges may be of some significance in the mediation of certain biologic properties of the immunoglobulins other than antigen binding.

Through enzyme degradation studies of the immunoglobulin molecule (Fig. 3-4), the antigen-binding portion (Fab) of the immunoglobulin was shown to consist of an L chain and a portion (Fd) of the H chain. Each monomeric unit of antibody globulin contains two such antigen-binding sites. When papain is used to cleave the immunoglobulin (IgG) molecule, two Fab fragments and one Fc portion per molecule result. However, when pepsin is used to treat the IgG molecule, the C_H2 portions of the heavy chains are degraded, leaving the C_H3 regions of the heavy chains and the $F(ab')_2$ fragment which contains the two antigen-binding sites of the intact molecule. Through utilization of the technic of affinity-labeling, Singer and Doolittle have shown that the affinity label (hapten antigen with chemically reactive side chain that forms covalent bonds with adjacent amino acids in the Fab sites after the hapten antigen has combined with antibody) binds

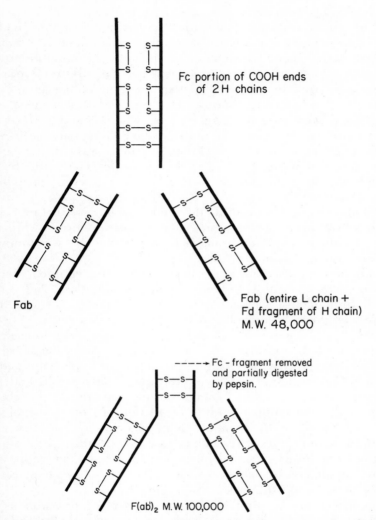

Fc portion of COOH ends
of 2 H chains

Fab

Fab (entire L chain +
Fd fragment of H chain)
M.W. 48,000

- - - → Fc - fragment removed
and partially digested
by pepsin.

F(ab)₂ M.W. 100,000

Fig. 3-4.—Immunoglobulin fragments resulting from enzymatic cleavage. *Top,* cleavage by papain. *Bottom,* cleavage by pepsin.

to both heavy and light chains in a ratio of about 2 to 1. Biologic properties other than antigen-binding are attributed to unique properties of the Fc region of the two H chains. The Fc portion also contains attached carbohydrate residues as depicted in Figure 3-3.

Intrachain disulfide bonds are regularly situated along each chain. Usually, two exist in each L chain and four are present in a gamma-type H chain. Occasionally, an additional bridge may be present in either a constant region (area of polypeptide chain containing a fairly constant sequence of amino acids) or variable region (areas of amino terminal ends of H and L chains containing highly variable amino acid sequence). Each bond encloses a loop consisting of 60–70 amino acids; these are referred to as domains. Examinations of the amino acid sequences of an immunoglobulin molecule around the cysteine of each bridge yield areas of homology, each of which contains about 110 amino acids. These are referred to as constant (C) regions. Little or no homology exists between these C regions and the variable (V) regions of the antigen-binding portion of the molecule. The sulfur for the disulfide bonds is provided by sulfur-containing amino acids (e.g., cysteine and methionine).

All light chains also exhibit this common basic structure which includes two intrachain disulfide bonds thereby forming the ring structures of the amino terminus (V region) and carboxy terminus (C region) of each L chain.

The immunoglobulin molecule has been subdivided into structural domains which exhibit different biologic activities. The immunoglobulin model of Edelman represented in Figure 3-3 shows these domains as does the model drawn in Figure 3-5. Regularly spaced disulfide-bridged loops of approximately 60 amino acids each are found along both the heavy and light chains. These loops are the domains and represent the V_L and C_L regions of the light chains and the V_H, C_H1, C_H2, and C_H3 regions of the heavy chains. IgE and IgM molecules appear to contain an extra loop on the heavy chains. Functionally, the antigen-binding (Fab) portions of each molecule consist of the V_L and V_H domains. Complement activation sites of the IgG and IgM molecules are contained in the C_H2 domain. On cytophilic antibody molecules, the attachment site for macrophages appears to be the C_H3 domain. Hay suggests that the binding of IgE to mast cells may be through its extra heavy chain domain.

Monomers and even dimers of L chains (Bence-Jones proteins) are found in the serum and urine of normal humans on occasion and more often in some patients with plasma cell dyscrasias such as multiple myeloma, agammaglobulinemia and systemic lupus erythematosus. Also, they are found in renal transplant patients and in the synovial fluids of patients with peripheral rheumatoid arthritis. Inter-light chain bonding often is found in Bence-Jones proteins which are commonly secreted as disulfide-bridged dimers. A possible explanation for the existence of these L chain units in the urine and serum of humans is the fact that an excess of L chains is needed for the syn-

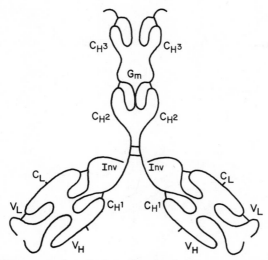

Fig. 3-5.—Diagram of an IgG molecule showing structural domains.

thesis of the whole immunoglobulin molecule or for reassembly of the isolated H and L chains. Moreover, L chains are catabolized in the kidney while H chains are not. Bence-Jones proteins exhibit the following characteristics: a molecular weight of 22,500 per single chain; a sedimentation coefficient in ultracentrifugal analysis of $S_{20w} = 3$–5S; and electrophoretic mobility in zone electrophoresis between that of a slow gamma-$_2$ globulin and an alpha-$_1$ globulin. They are reversibly precipitable between 40° and 60° C. This property is used diagnostically in the examination of human urine, especially in cases of multiple myeloma. If the precipitate which formed below 60° C dissolves during boiling and reforms on cooling, the specimen is positive for Bence-Jones proteins.

IgM molecules contain five monomeric units (i.e., a pentamer) joined by disulfide bonds which may be broken by mild reduction. Electronmicroscopic studies of IgM have revealed that the molecule is a circular polymer of five Y-shaped units as depicted in Figure 3-6, C. Flexibility of each Y-shaped monomer is thought to occur so that each unit may bend either above or below the plane of the circle. Each molecule contains 10 antigen-binding sites but only five of these seem to bind antigen well, although the other five do bind antigen.

IgA in serum may exist as a monomeric unit or as polymers (Fig. 3–6, A), e.g., dimers, trimers, pentamers or even larger structures. Secretory IgA is found in the conjunctiva, mouth, nasopharynx, gastrointestinal

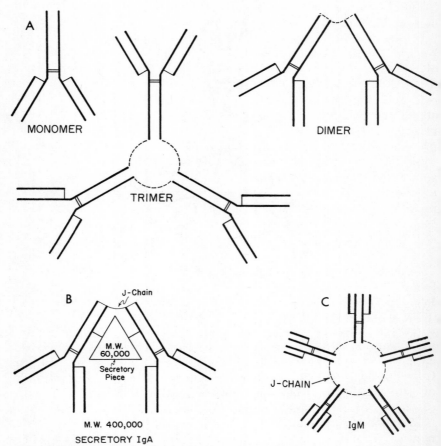

Fig. 3-6.—Polymeric and monomeric immunoglobulins. **A**, monomer, dimer and trimer, serum IgA. **B**, secretory IgA. **C**, IgM.

tract and urinary bladder. It is also found in breast milk and sweat. The secretory component (secretory piece, Fig. 3–6, B) is a single peptide chain with a molecular weight of about 60,000 to 70,000, contains about 6% carbohydrate and is produced by epithelial cells. In secretory IgA the secretory piece is bound to the carboxy terminal ends of the alpha chains via noncovalent bonds (and possibly by disulfide bonds). In the human (but not the rabbit) the secretory piece is bound to alpha chains by disulfide bonds. The secretory piece does not bear any close structural relationship to the immunoglobulins. It is even present in agammaglobulinemic humans who lack detectable amounts of either serum or secretory IgA.

The J (joining piece) chains are associated with polymeric immunoglobulin structures, IgM and IgA. The primary structure of the J-chain is not established, but it is rich in half-cysteine residues. The J-chain contains about 10% carbohydrate and has a molecular weight of approximately 20,000. The exact location of the J-chain in relation to the IgM and IgA molecules is uncertain. It is presumed to stabilize the polymeric forms of immunoglobulins in some manner, possibly by attaching covalently by a disulfide bond to an intersubunit bridge. It is present in a ratio of one J-chain per pentamer of whole IgM. It is not present in the Fab portion of human IgM.

Similar to IgG, the IgD and IgE immunoglobulins appear to exist as simple monomeric units of immunoglobulin. IgD molecules are labile to storage, perhaps due to their extreme sensitivity to digestion by the proteolytic enzymes of serum.

ALLOTYPIC MARKERS OF HUMAN IMMUNOGLOBULINS

In the human, three sets of allotypic markers on the immunoglobulin polypeptide chains are inherited. Within the IgG class, IgG_1 contains Gm allotypic antigens on both the Fc region and the constant portion of the Fd region of the H chains. Gm markers are found only in the Fc region of the IgG_2 and IgG_3 subclasses. No Gm markers have been identified on IgG_4. The Gm antigens are considered to be unique amino acids in the peptide chains and not carbohydrate in nature. Currently, these Gm markers number 25, some of which are distinctive of a given IgG subclass while others are not. Different ethnic groups display characteristic Gm factors.

Kappa light chains, present on all five classes of human immunoglobulins, display three (possibly four) allotypic markers located in the constant portion of the L chains. These are designated InV. The InV 1 and 2 markers are associated with leucine at amino acid position 191 and InV 3 is associated with valine at the same position. The Oz markers on lambda chains are isotypic markers present in all humans. Different lambda chains within the same individual may be displayed on different immunoglobulin molecules.

The allotypic markers are not readily detected serologically on either isolated H or L chains. Detection of these allotypes appears to require the presence of the antigen in the three-dimensional conformation of the entire immunoglobulin molecule.

The Am allotype marker is located on the alpha-2 chain of IgA_2. This system is genetically closely linked to that of the Gm system, but both are inherited independently of the kappa chain InV antigens. IgA_2 alpha chains are characterized as being Am 1 positive or Am 1 negative. Am 1 positive alpha-2 chains apparently lack disulfide bonds between the H and L chains while Am 1 negative molecules contain such disulfide bridges.

THEORIES OF ANTIBODY FORMATION

At the beginning of this century, Ehrlich postulated that antibodies are produced by a selective process. According to this concept, the mechanism for antibody production was present in an individual and antigen merely activated the process. Antigen selectively interacted with cells possessing receptors ("amboceptors") for antigen. Amboceptors (antibody-like substances) were present on cell surfaces. When antigens were present they bound to the specific amboceptors causing the amboceptors to be shed from the cell surface into the serum. Cells rapidly regenerated amboceptors under these conditions. (This process is remarkably similar to that which has recently been shown to occur.)

Then, for many years, from the early 1920's to the late 1950's, theoreticians postulated instructional models of antibody synthesis. Briefly, these are as follows. In the direct template model, antigen acted as a template around which the peptides of the globulin molecule were folded during antibody synthesis leaving the "imprint" of the antigenic determinants in all globulin molecules made in such cells. However, detectable antigen was never found in cells that were synthesizing antibody globulin. The indirect template theory of antibody formation again required that antigen serve as template but for an enzyme or enzyme systems which, in turn, instructed the folding of the antibody globulin for specific complementary fit with antigen. Again, no such enzymes were ever found.

Jerne was perhaps the first to revive the concept that selective processes are actually involved in antibody formation. Burnet in his postulates involving the clonal selection of antibody formation helped to turn attention once more to selective theories of antibody formation. The myriad of cells possessing receptors to all antigens to which an individual may eventually respond is present during fetal life. Cells reactive with self antigens are supposedly destroyed during fetal development and thereby are called "forbidden" clones. Individuals with autoimmune diseases are people in whom this destruction of "forbidden" clones did not occur properly. Burnet's prediction of immunologic tolerance to self antigens was later proved to exist in inbred animals made tolerant to allografts.

In more recent years, two schools of thought have existed to explain the expression of antibody production based on the fact that the

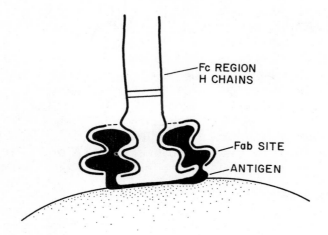

Fc REGION
H CHAINS

Fab SITE

ANTIGEN

Fig. 3-7.—Binding of antigenic determinants and immunoglobulin Fab sites.

capacity to elicit an immune response is a heritable characteristic. One such concept maintains that somatic mutation of genes is responsible for immunoglobulin production. This may explain the capacity of an individual to form antibodies to a wide array of antigens. However, the question remains unanswered as to exactly how all necessary mutations occur so as to afford an efficient immune responsiveness in a normal individual. A more compelling argument against this concept is that no known evidence of the occurrence of somatic mutations exists in mammals.

The second concept used to explain the selective process of antibody formation is called the germ line theory. According to this concept, all genes are present in an individual to specify the various classes and subclasses of immunoglobulins as well as the capability of forming antibodies to a wide variety of antigens. Recent evidence supports this concept. At least two genes control the synthesis of a single polypeptide chain of an immunoglobulin molecule. The constant regions for each class of immunoglobulin H chains may be specified by one gene for each class. Following the amino acid sequence determinations of isolated immunoglobulin polypeptide chains of monoclonal IgM, IgA or IgG classes (including each IgG subclass), the variable regions of the H chains were classified into four subgroups. Myeloma proteins are homogenous immunoglobulins produced by clones of malignant cells (cells descended from a single progenitor). They possess individually specific antigenic determinants (*idiotypes*) in the Fab region. Antibody molecules of a given idiotypic specificity are thought to be made by a single clone of cells. Consequently, by using human and mouse myeloma proteins, rabbit antibodies to bacterial antigens and a chick embryo B cell system, various investigators have shown that cells producing immunoglobulins of a given idiotype may also start to produce an immunoglobulin of the same idiotype but of another H chain class. For example, Wang and associates showed that a myeloma cell culture from a patient initially producing IgM eventually produced IgG of the same idiotype. In this system a genetic switching mechanism was postulated to have occurred. Further substantiation of this mechanism was provided by Penn and associates who observed a myeloma patient with two separable monoclonal serum proteins, IgG and IgA, of the same idiotype. Thus, a genetic switching mechanism may exist and may involve classes of immunoglobulin production other than IgM and IgG. Nisonoff and collaborators have speculated that idiotypic specificity may actually specify the antigen-binding (Fab) portion of the immunoglobulin molecule; i.e., all antibody molecules binding a given antigenic configuration to the same degree (e.g., a high affinity precise fit) may be identical in amino acid sequence, secondary and tertiary conformations and idiotypic specificity. To visualize this, imagine the variable portions of the L and H chains in the antibody combining sites depicted in Figure 3–7 existing on all classes and subclasses of immunoglobulins.

ANTIBODY PRODUCTION

The study of antibody production following injection of antigen by a parenteral route usually involves an evaluation of the serum antibodies that are produced. The serum is examined for its capacity to react specifically with antigen. In about 6 days after the initial injection of antigen (primary immunization), the first antibody detected in the serum is usually a 19S (IgM) globulin. By 10–14 days after antigen injection, the antibody activity is mainly associated with the 7S serum globulins (Fig. 3–8). Such 7S globulins consist mainly of IgG but may also contain some monomeric IgA. If a second injection of the same antigen (booster injection) is given at a later date, very little increase, if any, is seen in the level of 19S antibody stimulated, but a marked increase in both the amount and combining quality of the 7S globulin reactivity for antigen is seen. This secondary immune response (*anamnestic response*) is provoked more quickly than, and remains elevated longer than, that seen in the primary immunization.

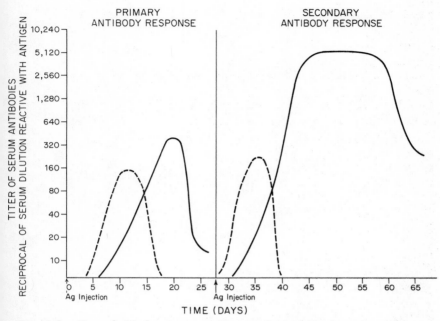

Fig. 3-8.—Hypothetical primary and secondary antibody responses. – – –
= 19S immunoglobulin (IgM); ——— = 7S immunoglobulins (mainly IgG).

Explanations for some of the differences between the primary and
secondary antibody responses now exist. Following primary immunization, the germinal centers of the lymphoid follicles increase in
number (Fig. 3–9). These areas are thought to contain specific B
lymphocytes in various stages of differentiation in response to antigen.
B lymphocytes on their way to becoming plasma cells appear to
migrate from the follicular areas to the area of the medullary cords in
the organized lymphoid tissue. The typical small lymphocyte contains
a relatively large nucleus in comparison to a small cytoplasmic mass.
The cytoplasm shows relatively few organelles. Upon stimulation by
antigen these cells show an increase in the amount of cytoplasm rich in
polysomes and rough endoplasmic reticulum. Some of these stimulated B cells differentiate into globulin-synthesizing and -secreting
plasma cells rich in rough endoplasmic reticulum and a well-
developed Golgi apparatus (Fig. 3–10). The carbohydrate residues are
attached to the H chains as the immunoglobulin molecules migrate
through the Golgi prior to secretion. Microscopic examinations have
revealed that globulins are secreted via vesicles formed in the Golgi

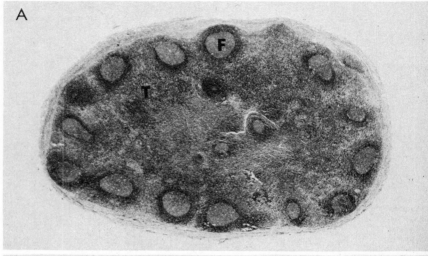

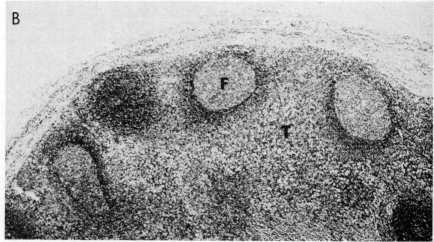

Fig. 3-9.—Cross-section of human lymph node. A, low power. B, high power. Numerous follicles (*F*) showing germinal centers (sites of B lymphocyte maturation). The paracortical thymus-dependent areas (*T*) are shown centrally.

apparatus in a process called *exocytosis* (the reverse of the endocytotic processes of pinocytosis and phagocytosis). In some plasma cells the cisternae of rough endoplasmic reticulum become distended with globulin and appear to burst, releasing the antibody into the surrounding medium (Fig. 3-11). Other stimulated B lymphocytes become B "memory cells" and eventually resemble small lymphocytes morphologically. Consequently, the number of antigen-specific B cells greatly increases following primary immunization. Using reagents (anti-H chain globulins) to localize immunoglobulins associated with lymphoid cells, various investigators have shown that each cell, at any one instance, is producing immunoglobulin molecules of only one H chain type. With anti-L chain reagents such cells seem always to produce immunoglobulins of the same L chain type. B cells exhibiting IgM receptors occur in the greatest numbers. Following antigenic stimulation, the B cells still exhibit a predominance of IgM and some cells exhibit IgG surface receptors. After the primary antibody response, the increased numbers of B memory cells obviously have immunoglobulin molecules on their membrane surfaces. Lymphoid cells in the process of becoming IgG-producing cells have been detected by using double labeling immunoglobulin reagents (e.g., rhodamine-conjugated anti-gamma chain and fluorescein-conjugated anti-mu chain sera). In this situation the cell surface receptors stain for IgM and the intracellular globulin being synthesized stains for IgG. Small lymphocytes (B cells) seem not to be the only cells capable of differentiating into plasma cells. Controversy over the origin of plasma cells exists. In an electronmicroscopic study, Kuhlmann and Avrameas have shown that both lymphocytes and reticulum cells can generate morphologically distinct plasma cells in rats immunized with horseradish peroxidase.

Upon secondary stimulation with antigen, the greater numbers of antigen-reactive B cells present are rapidly activated, accounting for the rapid increase in the serum of specific 7S antibody globulins. Examination of lymphoid tissues at this point reveals a greater number of plasma cells in the areas of the medullary cores as compared with the number seen after primary immunization. The antibody globulins produced during the anamnestic response are of higher binding quality (high affinity) than those produced during the primary immunization. Varying affinities of antibodies are produced during immunization. Usually, when an animal is initially immunized against a hapten, the earliest antibodies formed exhibit lower association constants (i.e., higher dissociation than binding rates) than those formed later. The reaction of antigen and antibody is a reversible union. High affinity antibodies exhibit a high degree of "fitting" to the complementary conformation of the antigenic groupings. Such antibodies exhibit high association constants, i.e., higher association rates as compared with rates of dissociation. Often a wide range of antibody affinities is seen at all stages of immunization. When the immunogen is a complex antigen, e.g., protein, the earliest antibodies are generally

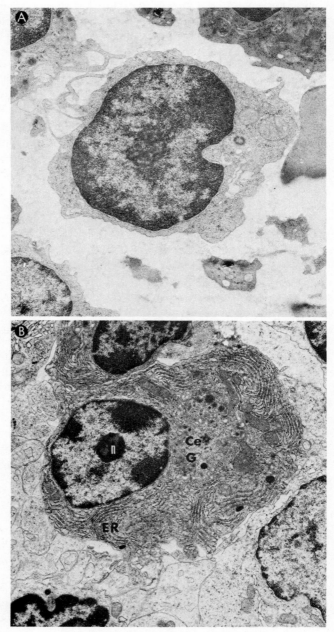

Fig. 3-10.—See legend on facing page.

not only of lower affinity but are also more highly selective for reaction with that particular antigen. Such antibodies cross-react little, if at all, even with closely related antigens. As immunization is repeated or prolonged, the antibodies not only exhibit a higher affinity for combination with the antigen (a better degree of fit), but also there seems to be a loss of selectivity. High affinity antibodies cross-react with related antigens but will not react with wholly unrelated antigens. A plausible explanation for this broadening of specificity is as follows. The first antibodies formed are directed against only a few of the different determinant groups of the antigen (the immunodominant groups). They are most likely the determinants most exposed in the tertiary structure of the antigen. The chance that these structures are the same as those on a related antigen is small. However, as immunization proceeds antibodies are formed against a larger proportion of the determinants of the "degraded" antigen. Thus, the antiserum contains a mixture of antibodies specific for a variety of different determinants, some of which are common to related antigen molecules. Consequently, the array of antibodies in an individual response to a given determinant can vary markedly in the strength with which they bind antigen. This depends upon minor alterations in the exactness of fit (or interlock) with the antigen.

Since cells bearing surface receptors which precisely fit the exposed antigenic groupings on the immunogen are able to bind antigen more firmly than cells bearing low affinity receptors, high affinity memory cells are selected out of the B cell population during primary immunization. Subsequently, when antigen is reintroduced the high affinity memory cells are rapidly activated to produce their high affinity product (immunoglobulin). Moreover, for similar reasons injections of small amounts of antigen stimulate high affinity antibodies while larger amounts of antigen stimulate the production of antibodies of lower affinities. Only those B cells with high affinity receptors will be able to bind sufficient antigen, when small amounts of antigen are present, for stimulation into antibody production. Thus, only high affinity antibody is produced. At higher antigen doses the B cells possessing lower affinity receptors will also be stimulated to produce antibody.

Fig. 3-10.—A, small lymphocyte. Electronmicrograph showing sparse cytoplasm with few organelles. **B,** plasma cell. Electronmicrograph showing eccentric nucleus with peripherally clumped chromatin (cartwheel appearance) and nucleolus (*n*). The abundant cytoplasm shows numerous lamellae of rough endoplasmic reticulum (*ER*) studded with ribosomes; a well-developed Golgi apparatus (*G*) surrounds a centriole (*Ce*).

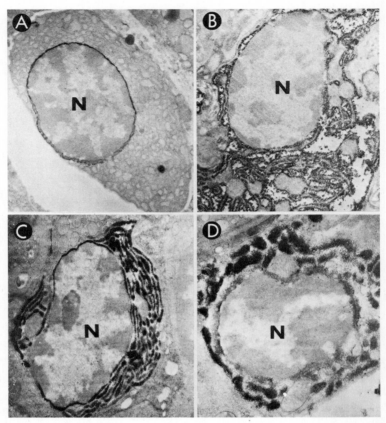

Fig. 3-11.—Antibody synthesis by plasma cells. An elegant and informative ultrastructural method of studying some of the intracellular events taking place in plasma cells during antibody synthesis has been devised using a plant enzyme, horseradish peroxidase, as an antigen which, when injected into experimental animals, elicits an immune response by producing antiperoxidase antibodies. After an appropriate period of time, the plasma cell-containing tissues of these animals are fixed in paraformaldehyde and exposed to a solution of peroxidase, so that the enzyme can bind to the antiperoxidase antibody in the cells. By appropriate cytochemical methods, an electron-dense amorphous precipitate may form at the site of enzyme activity and, hence, at the site of its antibody. After conventional processing, the tissue is examined unstained with the electron microscope for the presence of antiperoxidase-antibody-secreting plasma cells. Four such cells are seen here (× 12,000). **A,** the first evidence of antibody secretion occurs within the perinuclear space between the two membranes of the nuclear envelope. **B,** the activity then spreads to the ribosomes lining the cisternae of rough endoplasmic reticulum and then **C,** to the cisternae themselves, which become distended with antibody, while **D,** the nuclear envelope appears to lose part of its activity.

The injection of antibody specific for antigen can suppress a primary immunization response. IgG is most efficient in suppressing antibody synthesis. As expected, high affinity antibody is more effective than low affinity antibody in this suppressive effect. This observation has been used in the suppression of the capability of Rh-negative mothers to form anti-Rh_o (D) antibodies. Within 48–72 hours after delivery of an Rh-positive infant, human anti-Rh_o (D) (RhoGAM) is administered to the Rh-negative mother. Women thus treated fail to immunize to fetal Rh_o (D) erythrocytes and consequently are able to bear infants undamaged by erythroblastosis fetalis. No definite proof exists to adequately explain this suppression of antibody synthesis. However, it is argued that a competition exists between the injected antibody and the B cell receptors for the antigen. Only cells with receptors of higher affinity than that of the injected antibody will be stimulated.

Roitt explains these observations as follows: "As immunization proceeds, only lymphocytes with higher affinity receptors can be triggered because the concentration of available antigen steadily falls and feedback inhibition by synthesized antibody will 'turn off' cells with equal or lower affinity receptors." He also compares the efficiency of IgM and IgG molecules in their relative abilities to bind antigen. Roitt distinguishes between affinity and avidity. *Affinity* describes the equilibrium reaction between the Fab sites on the immunoglobulins and the antigenic determinants. *Avidity* applies to the reactions between whole molecules of immunoglobulins and antigens. In this context the valence of antigens is highly significant. In the comparison of IgM and IgG molecules of equal affinities for a given antigen, the IgM molecules would exert a greater avidity for the antigen because of its 10 antigen-binding sites. Consequently, B cells with IgM surface receptors of lower affinity than B cells with IgG receptors of high affinity may bind the same number of antigen molecules.

IMMUNOGLOBULIN LEVELS

In Table 3-2 various values pertaining to immunoglobulin metabolism are shown. Of all the various classes of immunoglobulins, note that the synthetic rate is the greatest and the catabolic rate is the least for IgG. Within the IgG class 70% of the serum IgG is of the IgG_1 subclass; 20% is of the IgG_2 subclass; 8–9% is of the IgG_3 subclass; approximately 1% is of the IgG_4 subclass. For an as yet unexplained reason, IgG_2 appears earlier in immunization than does the IgG_1 (IgG_2 is slower electrophoretically than IgG_1).

The importance of the IgG class of antibodies, especially in antimicrobial immunity and in the passive transfer of immune serum

TABLE 3-2.—IMMUNOGLOBULIN LEVELS

CHARACTERISTIC	IMMUNOGLOBULIN CLASS				
	IgM	IgG	IgA	IgD	IgE
Serum level					
mg/ml	$0.3–1 \pm 0.75$	$10–18.2 \pm 4.53$	$0.73–3.94 \pm 0.91$	0.03	*
mg/100 ml	50–200	700–1500	100–400	0.3–0.4	
Half-life (days)	2	20–25	6–7	2.8	
		$(IgG_3, 7.5–9)$			
Synthetic rate (mg/kg/day)	7	35	25	0.4	
Catabolism: intravascular					
pool (%/day)	18	6.8	25	37	
Age at which adult level reached (years)	$\frac{1}{2}–1$	2	8–12		15–20*

*In nonatopic (normal) individuals, "normal serum levels" = 0.1–0.7 µM/ml.

56

either naturally via the placenta or artificially by parenteral injection, is supported by the fact that the half-life of three of the subclasses is 20–25 days. This is approximately 3 times longer than that of IgG$_3$ or any of the other classes of immunoglobulins. Even though IgA is synthesized at rates approaching that of IgG, it is catabolized at about 4 times the rate of IgG. Immunoglobulin light chains are catabolized in the kidneys, but the sites of catabolism of the heavy chains and the intact immunoglobulin molecules are, as yet, unknown.

Note that IgM is present only in small amounts in internal secretions. It, as well as IgE, may be produced locally in the lamina propria of mucous membranes of glandular tissue. In humans deficient in IgA production, a compensatory increase in the IgM content of body secretions appears. Small amounts of IgG appear in body secretions normally. Tomasi cites a ratio for IgG:IgA of 0.01 (1 IgG:100 IgA) in parotid saliva compared with 4–5 (4–5 IgG:IgA) for serum. The IgG, IgE and most IgM in secretory fluids appear identical to those molecules present in serum, while about one tenth of the IgM in body secretions has a "secretory component" attached.

Adult levels of immunoglobulins are reached at various times. Only three of the four IgG subclasses of immunoglobulins pass the placenta in fetal life; IgG$_2$ appears unable to pass through the placenta. Consequently, at birth the human infant is not only protected by maternal antibodies against a variety of microbial parasites but also is suppressed immunologically by the 7S antibody feedback mechanism. Even though the T lymphocyte system is capable of functioning at birth or even in the fetus, some doubt has existed as to whether the B cell or macrophage systems are adequately mature at birth to insure a vigorous antibody response. Recently data concerning the capabilities of the human fetus to produce antibodies have accumulated. In spite of the existence of maternal antibodies which no doubt do suppress the fetal response to antigens, upon infection of the fetus with certain viruses (e.g., measles or lymphocytic choriomeningitis viruses against which the mother was not previously protected) the fetus is able to mount an antibody response. Serum IgM is detected upon birth in such infants and certain investigators feel that the fetal production of IgG$_2$ should be evaluated, also. In the tears of neonates infected in utero, IgA is detected within days of birth in contrast to healthy uninfected newborn infants who usually first demonstrate IgA in tears at about 21 days of life.

Adult levels are reached within $1/2$–1 year for IgM, by 2 years for IgG, and sometime between the age of 8 to 12 years for IgA. In nonallergic individuals adult levels of IgE seem to be reached sometime between 15 to 20 years of life, while atopic individuals demon strate higher levels of IgE earlier. Little is known about the age at which adult levels of IgD occur. However, recent evidence indicates that IgD may be of significance in the human fetus (see Chapter 7).

The newborn human is especially prone to infections by gram-negative enteric bacilli. Most human antibody produced against the endotoxins of these bacilli is mainly of the IgM class; since the only protection present in the neonate is the maternal IgG the infant must acquire its own immune experience against bacterial endotoxins. IgA antibodies against *E. coli* were present in colostrum-fed human infants who were more resistant to attacks of diarrhea than were infants not fed colostrum. South has postulated that the maternal IgA in colostrum is adsorbed onto the infant's intestinal mucosa, remains there resisting the digestive processes and protects the infant against gram-negative enteric bacilli. Secretory IgA (with the secretory component attached) appears more resistant to enzyme digestion than do all of the serum immunoglobulins. Since IgA molecules lack a complement attachment site, these antibodies are probably not responsible for bacteriolytic destruction of the enteric bacilli with the subsequent liberation of endotoxin and other toxic bacterial products onto the surface of the mucosa. They probably function as opsonins and aid in the phagocytic uptake of the bacteria.

BIOLOGIC FUNCTIONS OF HUMAN IMMUNOGLOBULINS

All five classes of human immunoglobulins function as antibodies. Biologic properties other than antigen-binding are associated with the Fc regions of the immunoglobulin H chains and are listed in Table 3-3. IgM is the first antibody made following parenteral injection of antigen. Because of its valence it is an efficient antibody molecule in certain in vitro tests (e.g., complement-fixation) and in various aspects of antimicrobial immunity. As a B cell receptor, IgM is obviously of significance in the initiation of the antibody response. IgG is the major serum globulin functioning in antimicrobial immunity. It is that portion of the maternal immune response which is transferred in utero via the placenta to the fetus and subsequently functions in an-timicrobial protection of the neonate for its first several months of life.

The significance of the IgA system of immunoglobulins as a key portion of the immune response is still evolving. The secretory IgA system appears to be an immune system distinctly separate from the systemic immune system. It seems to be a local immune system associated with the mucous membranes, conjunctiva and body secre-

TABLE 3-3.—BIOLOGIC FUNCTIONS OF HUMAN IMMUNOGLOBULINS

BIOLOGIC FUNCTION	IMMUNOGLOBULINS INVOLVED
Antibody activity	IgM, IgG, IgA, IgD, IgE
Serum antibody	Mainly IgG; also IgM and IgA
Host protection: Mucous membranes and conjunctiva	Mainly IgA; some IgM and IgG
Placental transfer	
Natural passive protection	IgG_1, IgG_3 and IgG_4
Complement-fixing site	1 type of IgM; IgG_1, IgG_3 (IgG_2 fixes complement poorly)

TABLE 3-4.—PATHOLOGIC COUNTERPARTS OF NORMAL IMMUNOGLOBULINS

PATHOLOGIC STATE	IMMUNOGLOBULIN INVOLVED
Atopy, anaphylactic type allergy	Mainly IgE (reagin, homocytotropic properties)
Multiple myelomas	Serum: Usually monoclonal spike of IgG, IgA, or IgE; occasionally diclonal Urine: L chain monomers and/or dimers (Bence-Jones proteins)
Waldenström's macroglobulinemia	Serum: Monoclonal spike of IgM Urine: Bence-Jones proteins
H chain diseases	Gamma, alpha or mu chain disease; H chains (corresponding to Fc regions) Serum: H chain pieces Urine: Mainly in IgG type H chain disease find H chain pieces

tions such as milk, saliva and tears. As discussed previously, the secretory piece of IgA is produced by epithelial cells and is present even in individuals lacking IgA-producing cells. Cells which produce secretory IgA are located in the lamina propria beneath the mucosal surface. Differences exist between not only levels of secretory and serum IgA but also among the levels of secretory IgA in various areas of mucosa. Although the main site of serum IgA synthesis is controversial, Tomasi cites evidence indicating that IgA generated in the gastrointestinal tract is able to enter the vascular compartment. Since 85% of circulating IgA in humans is in monomeric form, that portion of IgA which enters the circulation from the gut probably diffuses into the vascular compartment as a 7S molecule. Even though plasma cells staining for IgA content are present in peripheral lymphoid tissues and are one-third to one-fourth as frequent as are cells producing IgG in these sites, the mucous membranes appear to be the main sites of IgA production. As yet, a quantitation of the transport of IgA molecules from mucosa to serum has not been established.

No aspect of vaccination procedures used in humans has been more revealing of the significance of secretory IgA than that of virus vaccines. When killed polio virus is injected into humans by a parenteral route, adequate levels of circulating serum antibodies result. But no antibody is present at either the route of entry (nasopharynx) or sites of initial infection (gastrointestinal tract) by the polio virus. However, when living, attenuated polio virus is introduced by a natural route of infection (orally), excellent secretory IgA responses develop in the nasopharynx and gut as well as do good levels of circulating antibodies. The story has repeated itself in immunization of humans with killed and living measles virus vaccines. This experience taught most pointedly the lesson that *the natural route of viral entry must be immunologically protected* to simulate the immunity developed from actually having had (and recovered from) an infectious disease. In children receiving killed measles virus parenterally, excellent antibody titers existed in the sera. When these children were subsequently infected naturally by the respiratory route with measles virus, the virus replicated in the cells of the unprotected lungs. Consequently, adequate amounts of virus were released into the circulation and, in some children, reacted with antibody (present in high titers) producing manifestations of immune complex disease (see Chapter 9). The plasma cells of the lamina propria and the IgA in secretions and serum seem to reach adult levels at about puberty. These levels increase rapidly during the first year of life and are first detectable at approximately 21 days. The lack or deficiency in IgA is associated with several genetic immunodeficiency diseases as well as with certain individuals who have developed autoimmune disease. These aspects of the IgA system are discussed further in Chapters 7 and 10 in relation to these diseases.

Currently, the normal biologic functions for both IgE and IgD have not been established. However, certain evidence indicates that IgE may play some role in protective immunity of the sinopulmonary tract to infectious disease agents and that IgD may be a significant fetal immunoglobulin.

Although suspected, it has been difficult to show directly that antibody plays a regulatory role in certain physiologic processes. Some evidence exists indicating that certain antibodies (autoantibodies) to self antigens may either protect cells (e.g., red cells from shearing forces in capillaries) or aid in the clearance of effete host cells and degradation products.

PATHOLOGIC COUNTERPARTS OF HUMAN IMMUNOGLOBULINS (TABLE 3-4)

Even though the normal function of IgE in the human is uncertain, its pathologic counterpart in atopic allergies is well documented. The predisposition toward atopy is inherited. In atopic individuals the Fab portion of the IgE molecule reacts with the *allergen* (antigen against which IgE response is directed). A peculiar property of the IgE is that the Fc regions of the epsilon chains of the molecule bind to certain cells, mast cells in particular. This property is utilized in demonstrations of the passive transfer of atopic reactivity to nonatopic individuals. Twenty-four hours following intradermal injection, the specific allergen-binding capacity of the serum is demonstrable when allergen is injected and a positive-skin test is evoked. The capacity of IgE to fix to cells in tissues is referred to as its *homocytotropic* property. When allergen interacts with IgE fixed to mast cells, the mast cells degranulate releasing vasoactive substances which are the actual mediators of the allergic reaction in the individual. This reaction is discussed further in Chapter 9.

The other pathologic counterparts of normal immunoglobulins are the "paraproteins" or "M-components" of the gammopathies. Most gammopathies appear to be the result of a malignant transformation of a B cell or its precursor.

Multiple Myelomas

Multiple myelomas are usually monoclonal gammopathies characterized by the appearance in the serum of one M-component which is an homogenous protein composed of a single type of immunoglobulin molecule. Such homogenous proteins are considered to be the product of the transformed cell and its daughter cells. Approximations of the various immunoglobulin classes of all human monoclonal gammopathies are: 54% are IgG; 20% are IgA; 16% are IgM; 8% are Bence-Jones. The remaining 2–3% are comprised of the IgE and IgD myelomas and the heavy chain type monoclonal gammopathies. Most of the structural studies done on the immunoglobulin molecules have been performed with the homogenous myeloma proteins. Were it not for myeloma proteins, structural studies of IgE and IgD molecules would not have been possible since they are present in normal individuals in extremely low amounts. Occasionally, diclonal myelomas have been found in the human. Multiple myelomas appear in later life, more frequently after 40 years of age, and seem to occur twice as frequently in males as in females. A monoclonal spike of the homogenous myeloma globulin appears in the gamma globulin region of the serum upon electrophoresis. In 40–50% of myeloma patients, Bence-Jones proteins are present and readily detected in the urine. The immunoglobulin class of the M-component may be identified by examining the patient's serum in an immunoelectrophoretic analysis (see Chapter 5).

Even though myeloma proteins have been used for structural studies of the immunoglobulin molecules, most such homogenous globulins appear to be intact molecules. Exceptions do exist, however. An IgG myeloma protein with a molecular weight of 120,000 has been identified in which the variable region of the Fd segment of the H chains was absent. Half molecules of immunoglobulins have been seen in multiple myeloma of mice. Only recently have half molecules of immunoglobulin been seen in a human myeloma patient. This particular case involved half molecules of IgA.

Patients with multiple myeloma display a defect in the capacity to make antibodies to new antigenic stimuli; i.e., a general defect in the activation of B lymphocytes. In such patients, T lymphocyte functions appear unhindered. The reason for the B cell deficiency in these patients is uncertain. Initially, the malignant B cells were thought to "crowd out" the normal B cell precursors in the bone marrow. More recently, RNA-containing serum factors (in the globulin fraction) have been found in mouse and human myelomas which seem to depress selectively the function of normal B cells while stimulating receptors on myeloma B cells. Also, another serum substance migrating electrophoretically as an alpha$_1$ globulin appears in the sera of some humans with malignant diseases and seems also to depress normal B cell function and possibly certain T cell functions. This substance is called immunoregulatory alpha globulin (IRA) or Mowbray factor.

Patients with multiple myeloma may exhibit anemia (normochromic anemia and usually low reticulocyte counts), multifocal bone pain, weight loss and, in rare instances, hepatosplenomegaly. Plasma cells are present in the bone marrow but are rarely found in the peripheral blood of myeloma patients. These patients have greatly elevated erythrocyte sedimentation rates.

Eight to 25 percent of all myelomas are merely light chain disease (Bence-Jones monoclonal myopathy) and are characterized by the detection of free light chains on immunoelectrophoresis of serum and urine. Also, a nonsecretory form of multiple myeloma exists in which no abnormal serum proteins are detected. Only plasmacytosis is seen. Characterization of this disease involves the detection of monoclonal-staining plasma cells in bone marrow specimens (using immunofluorescent reagents which are H chain-specific as well as separate reagents which are L chain-specific). *Waldenström's macroglobulinemia* is a chronic neoplastic disease of the bone marrow with monoclonal IgM being the product of the neoplastic cells. Microscopically these cells may look like either plasma cells or lymphocytes. This disease is clinically similar to chronic lymphatic leukemia and occurs mainly in individuals over 50 years of age. Such patients may exhibit anemia either with or without weight loss. In contrast to patients with multiple myeloma, those with Waldenström's macroglobulinemia commonly have hepatosplenomegaly and generalized lymphadenopathy but rarely have osteolytic bone lesions. Also, pancytopenia and granulocytopenia with relative lymphocytosis occur. Hemorrhagic purpura is seen especially involving the mucous membranes. As the disease progresses, the increased serum viscosity resulting from increased levels of IgM often leads to circulatory problems and heart failure. Moreover, because of the size of the IgM, kidney involvement is also seen. In 10% of macroglobulinemia patients, Bence-Jones proteinuria is detected. Detection of a monoclonal spike of IgM (macroglobulin) in the serum of these patients by electrophoresis and immunoelectrophoresis aids in the diagnosis.

H Chain Diseases

The H chain diseases may appear secondary to a primary malignancy involving lymphoid tissue. To date, three types of H chain disease have been identified: gamma chain disease, alpha chain disease and mu chain disease. Franklin predicts that delta and epsilon chain diseases will be found eventually.

GAMMA CHAIN DISEASE.—The gamma chain disease (Franklin's disease) has been seen in middle-aged or elderly individuals. Since patients exhibit lymphadenopathy, disease is characterized clinically as a malignant lymphoma. These patients undergo repeated febrile episodes and usually die of infection. By electrophoretic examination, their sera and urine contain a broad protein peak migrating in the beta globulin region. The urinary protein does not show the thermal precipitating properties of Bence-Jones proteins. Such abnormal protein components possess sedimentation coefficients of 3.5–4S and are actually portions of the H chain dimers of the IgG molecule. These fragments react with antiserum directed against the Fc region of the IgG molecule; i.e., they react with anti-gamma chain sera and not with either anti-kappa or anti-lambda chain sera. The amino acid sequences of several abnormal H chain components have been determined. In one such study, the H chains of an IgG_3 molecule were found to contain a deletion of amino acid constituents from position 19 at the N-terminus to amino acid position 216 near the hinge region. The region of deletion includes a major portion of the variable region of the Fd segment of each H chain. This appears to be the region deleted in several other gamma chain disease molecules. Thus, the H chain dimers in gamma chain disease appear to be composed of the Fc region and a small portion of the Fd segment of the H chains. Usually, no L chains have been detected in cells that are producing the abnormal H chains. Possibly the gene(s) controlling the variable regions of the L and H chains have been deleted or repressed in the malignant transformation of these cells. However, one patient with a gamma chain disease did exhibit Bence-Jones proteinuria.

ALPHA CHAIN DISEASE.—Abnormal alpha chain production is associated with malignant lymphomas involving the gastrointestinal tract, normally the major site of IgA synthesis. When first described alpha chain disease occurred in people of Mediterranean origins. Subsequently, the occurrence of this abnormality has been observed in people from South America and other parts of Europe. This disease exhibits a rapid clinical course. Patients show malabsorption, diarrhea, weight loss and cachexia. Other than in the gastrointestinal tract, the lymphoid organs show little involvement in alpha chain disease. The sera of these patients do not exhibit any marked abnormalities upon electrophoresis. Moreover, the urine of the patients contains very little of the abnormal H chains, possibly because of the tendency of alpha chains to form dimers, trimers, etc.

MU CHAIN DISEASE.—Mu chain abnormalities have been observed in three patients with longstanding chronic lymphocytic leukemia. In mu chain disease, the patient's bone marrow contains vacuolated plasma cells that are rarely seen in other diseases. The content of the vacuoles is not known, but Franklin has observed that it is not protein. Two of the three patients studied excreted large amounts of kappa-type light chains into the urine. Using rhodamine-labeled anti-mu chain serum and anti-kappa chain serum labeled with fluorescein isothiocyanate, the plasma cells of the three patients were examined. In only one of these instances were both mu and kappa chains present in the same cell. No H chains are excreted in the urine in this disease. The mu chain abnormality is difficult to detect in electrophoretic examinations of serum and urine. Not only are the abnormal mu chains absent in the urine, but the serum electrophoretic patterns appear normal. However, when one such serum was examined by immunoelectrophoresis, a rapidly migrating band (molecular weight approximately 55,000) was found reactive only with anti-mu chain and not reactive with either anti-kappa or anti-lambda chain sera. One of these patients also had amyloid associated with the mu chain disease. The significance of this observation is unclear.

Zawadzki and Edwards have classified the human monoclonal immunoglobulin disorders into three categories: malignant immunocytopathy with monoclonal immunoglobulinemia, nonmyelomatous monoclonal immunoglobulinemia, and pseudoparaproteinemia. Within the malignant immunocytopathies, they have included multiple myeloma, Waldenström's macroglobulinemia, lichen myxedematosus, malignant lymphoma, heavy chain diseases, monocytic leukemia and amyloidosis.

Amyloidosis frequently appears associated with lymphoreticular disorders. Franklin and Zucker-Franklin suggest that amyloid occurs when the antigenic stimulation is excessive for the available immune system. When amyloid is associated with malignancy, they offer the suggestion that its formation has escaped the normal control mechanisms because of the neoplastic change. Certain amyloid fibrils (molecular weight of 5,000–18,300) are composed of the variable regions of immunoglobulin light chains. Lambda chains are associated with the amyloid paraproteins twice as frequently as are kappa chains. Also, proteins containing amino acid sequences different from those of immunoglobulin light chains have been identified in certain amyloid fibrils. Certain cases of amyloidosis occur in the absence of any known associated disease and are called primary amyloidosis. In these instances, amyloid deposits are found in the mesodermal tissues (smooth and skeletal muscle) and/or in the cardiovascular system. Secondary amyloidosis is associated with chronic disorders such as infections, connective tissue diseases or malignancies. Franklin and Zucker-Franklin have observed that the distribution of amyloid associated with multiple myeloma resembles that of primary amyloidosis. The amyloid associated with solid tumors is typified by deposits in tissues such as skin, respiratory tract and bladder. Also, many cases of familial types of amyloidosis have been described.

Other Immunoglobulin Abnormalities

Other types of monoclonal immunoglobulinemias occur in humans, but their clinical significance is not well understood. In infants and young children, monoclonal immunoglobulinemia is usually limited to those with immunodeficiency states. Paraproteinemia may be transient or associated with autoimmune or malignant diseases. Nonmyelomatous monoclonal immunoglobulinemia has been associated with cirrhosis of the liver, drug allergies and chronic infections.

Zawadzki and Edwards point out that any component present in human serum or plasma in excess of 300 mg per 100 ml may be detected as an identifiable spike in the electropherogram. Normally, only albumin and fibrinogen exceed this limit. However, pseudoparaproteins are seen occasionally in sera with a high titer of rheumatoid factor or in sera containing high concentrations of lipoproteins, hemoglobin or contaminated with bacterial products.

Apparently, any region of an immunoglobulin molecule may be deleted in malignant processes involving antibody-producing cells. De Coteau and associates have described a monoclonal protein in the serum and urine of a patient with a lymphoma resembling Hodgkin's disease. This monoclonal protein was the $F(ab')_2$ fragment of an IgM molecule and was designated as $F(ab')_2$. Also, intact 7S monomeric subunits of IgM have been described in multiple myeloma, lymphomas, systemic lupus erythematosus and hereditary telangiectasia.

SUGGESTED READINGS

Anfinsen, C. B.: Principles that govern the folding of protein chains, Science 181:223, 1973.

Burnet, F. M.: *Cellular Immunology* (Carlton: Melbourne University Press; London: Cambridge University Press, 1969).

Burnet, F. M., and Fenner, F.: *The Production of Antibodies* (2nd ed.; Melbourne: MacMillan, 1949).

Buxbaum, J. N.: The biosynthesis, assembly, and secretion of immunoglobulin, Semin. Hematol. 10:33, 1973.

Conway, B. P.: Technical aspects of the detection and characterization of immunoglobulin dyscrasias, Health Lab. Sci. 9:185, 1972.

De Coteau, W. E., Calvanico, N. J., and Tomasi, T. B., Jr.: Malignant lymphoma with a multiclonal F(ab)μ fragment, Clin. Immunol. Immunopathol. 1:190, 1973.

Dettlebach, H. R., and Ritzmann, S. E.: Lab Synopsis, Diagnostic Reagents Bulletin, Vol. 2, (2nd ed.; New York: Behring Diagnostics, 1969).

Edelman, G. M.: The structure and function of antibodies, Sci. Am. 223:34, 1970.

Edelman, G. M.: Antibody structure and molecular immunology, Ann. N.Y. Acad. Sci. 190:5, 1971.

Frangione, B., and Franklin, E. C.: Heavy chain diseases: clinical features and molecular significance of the disordered immunoglobulin structure, Semin. Hematol. 10:53, 1973.

Franklin, E. C.: Some Protein Disorders Associated with Neoplasms of Plasma Cells and Lymphocytes: Heavy Chain Diseases, in Amos, B. (ed.): Progress in Immunology I (New York: Academic Press, 1971), p. 745.

Franklin, E. C., and Frangione, B.: The molecular defect in a protein (CRA) found in γ 1 heavy chain disease, and its genetic implications, Proc. Nat. Acad. Sci. U.S.A. 68:187, 1971.

Franklin, E. C., and Zucker-Franklin, D.: Current concepts of amyloid, Adv. Immunol. 15:249, 1972.

Fudenberg, H. H., Pink, J. R. L., Stites, D. P., and Wang, A-C.: Basic Immunogenetics (London: Oxford University Press, 1972).

Glenner, G. G., Terry, W. D., and Isersky, C.: Amyloidosis: its nature and pathogenesis, Semin. Hematol. 10:65, 1973.

Hay, F. C.: Effector sites associated with immunoglobulin domains, Current Titles Immunol. Transplant. and Allergy 1:484, 1973.

Jerne, N. K.: The natural selection theory of antibody formation, Proc. Nat. Acad. Sci. U.S.A. 41:849, 1955.

Kochwa, S., and Kunkel. H. G. (eds.): Immunoglobulins, Ann. N.Y. Acad. Sci. 190, 1971.

Kuhlmann, W. D., and Avrameas, S.: Cellular differentiation and antibody localization during the primary immune response in peroxidase stimulated lymph nodes of rat, Cell. Immunol. 4:425, 1972.

Maddison, S. E.: Structure and function of human immunoglobulins, Health Lab. Sci. 9:167, 1972.

Nisonoff, A., et al.: Genetic Control of the Biosynthesis of IgG and IgM, in Amos, B. (ed.): Progress in Immunology I (New York: Academic Press, 1971), p. 61.

Penn, G. M., Kunkel, H. G., and Grey, H. M.: Sharing of individual antigenic determinants between a γ G and a γ M protein in the same myeloma serum, Proc. Soc. Exp. Biol. Med. 135:660, 1970.

Porter, R. R.: Structural studies of immunoglobulins, Science 180:713, 1973.

Potter, M.: The developmental history of the neoplastic plasma cell in mice: A brief review of recent developments, Semin. Hematol. 10:19, 1973.

Putnam, F. W., et al.: Complete amino acid sequence of the mu heavy chain of a human IgM immunoglobulin, Science 182:287, 1973.

Reimer, C. B.: Standardization of immunoglobulin reagents, Health Lab. Sci. 9:178, 1972.

Ritzmann, S. E., Daniels, J. C., and Lawrence, M. C.: Monoclonal gammopathies: Present status, Texas Med. 68:91, 1972.

Roitt, I.: Essential Immunology (Oxford: Blackwell Scientific Publications, 1971).

Rowe, D. S., et al.: IgD on the surface of peripheral blood lymphocytes of the human newborn, Nat. New Biol. 242:155, 1973.

Singer, S. J., and Doolittle, R. F.: Antibody active sites and immunoglobulin molecules, Science 153:13, 1966.

Solomon, A., and McLaughlin, C. L.: Immunoglobulin structure determined from products of plasma cell neoplasms, Semin. Hematol. 10:3, 1973.

South, M. A.: IgA in neonatal immunity, Ann. N. Y. Acad. Sci. 176:40, 1971.

Tomasi, T. B.: Human immunoglobulin A, N. Engl. J. Med. 279:1327, 1968.

Tomasi, T. B.: Secretory immunoglobulins, N. Engl. J. Med. 287:500, 1972.

Wang, A-C, et al.: Evidence for control of synthesis of the variable regions of the heavy chains of IgG and IgM by the same gene, Proc. Nat. Acad. Sci. U.S.A. 66:337, 1970.

Yunginger, J. W., and Gleich, G. J.: Seasonal changes in serum and nasal IgE concentrations, J. Allergy Clin. Immunol. 51:174, 1973.

Zawadzki, Z. A., and Edwards, G. A.: Nonmyelomatous monoclonal immunoglobulinemia, Prog. Clin. Immunol. 1:105, 1972.

4 / Complement

The complement system consists of eleven plasma proteins (C1q, C1r, C1s, C2, C3, C4, C5, C6, C7, C8 and C9). The biologic significance of this complex system puzzled investigators for years. Since its participation in the in vitro complement-fixation test (the binding of certain complement components to the Fc region of certain antibody globulins whose Fab regions are bound to antigen) has been widely used serologically, involvement of the complement system in in vivo immunologic reactions was suspected but not proven until recently. Once activated, the reaction sequence and products of the complement components act as effectors in the inflammatory response.

Components of the complement system are serum glycoproteins of varying molecular weights (79,000 to 400,000 daltons). The sedimentation coefficients of the complement components vary between 4S and 10S except for the C1 complex (C1qrs), which has a sedimentation coefficient of 19S. The C1q portion of the C1 complex exhibits a sedimentation coefficient of 11S. Electrophoretically, C1q and C8 are gamma globulins; C1r, C2, C3, C4, C5, C6 and C7 are beta globulins; and C1s and C9 are alpha globulins. The complexity of this system is exemplified by observations that certain of these components are not homogenous proteins. Actually, C3 is composed of two components which migrate in an electric field as a beta globulin (β_1A) and an alpha$_2$ globulin (α_2D). C9 migrates electrophoretically in the alpha$_2$ to alpha$_1$ region.

The sites of synthesis of complement remain obscure. C3 and C6 components are seemingly synthesized in the liver; the C1 complex (C1qrs) appears to be synthesized in the small intestine; C4 is made by the macrophages of the reticuloendothelial system in guinea pigs; C2 appears to be made in large mononuclear cells of lymphoid tissues, lung and peritoneal exudates.

ACTIVATION OF CLASSIC COMPLEMENT PATHWAY

The complement system may be activated by complexes of antigen and antibody (IgM, IgG$_1$, IgG$_2$ or IgG$_3$) or by aggregated human immunoglobulins. The classic complement reaction sequence ("cascade") is shown in Figure 4-1. This scheme has been established by studying the lysis of sheep erythrocytes (SRBC's) in the presence of rabbit antibody (anti-SRBC). Activation of the complement "cascade" is initiated by the binding of the C1q subunit of the first component, C1, to the immunoglobulin Fc region of the antibody-antigen complex. In the inactive state the C1s of the C1 complex is bound to an $alpha_2$ globulin (the $C\bar{1}$ inhibitor). Otherwise the active $C\bar{1}$ complex is either bound to antigen-antibody or free in the serum as $C\bar{1}$ is esterolytic through the $C\bar{1}s$ component. Calcium (Ca^{++}) is essential for the formation of an active first component of complement ($C\bar{1}$ esterase). Once the $C\bar{1}$ esterase activity exists, C4 is cleaved into at least two portions. The larger C4 fragment either adheres to antigenic sites on the erythrocyte or remains hemolytically inactive in the surrounding fluid. Then $C\bar{1}$ rapidly cleaves C2. These reactions are catalyzed by magnesium ion. The portions of C4 and C2 which are attached to the antigen-antibody unit are designated as $C\overline{4\text{-}2}$ and function as a convertase enzyme for complement component C3. At this point in the reaction sequence many C3 units may be activated and funneled into the reaction. C3 is cleaved into two fragments, the larger of which may either bind to the cellular antigen or remain inactive in the fluid phase. The cellular attachment of $C\bar{3}$ then creates a complex (consisting of antigen-antibody-$C\overline{1423}$) that exhibits a new enzyme activity which then cleaves C5. The major fragment of $C\bar{5}$ is bound to the complex and $C\bar{6}$ is rapidly added. After the addition of $C\bar{7}$ to the growing complex, the cellular intermediate is stable and capable of reacting with C8 and C9. Upon addition of the $C\bar{8}$ and $C\bar{9}$ components, the erythrocyte membrane is structurally altered and hemoglobin is lost to the fluid phase.

During the complement reaction "cascade" enhancement of the inflammatory response occurs. The antigen-antibody-C (Ag-Ab$C\bar{1}$) and Ag-Ab$C\overline{1423}$ complexes exhibit immune adherence by sticking to phagocytic cells and thereby facilitate phagocytic ingestion. Human monocytes have surface receptors for not only C1 and C3 but also for IgM and IgG. Moreover, B lymphocytes have surface receptor areas for C3. Low molecular weight peptides split from the C3 and C5 components and not bound in the complement cascade reactions are designated as C3a and C5a. Both C3a and C5a peptides exhibit anaphylatoxin activity (enhance vascular permeability, stimulate contraction of smooth muscle and provoke the release of histamine from mast cells). The C5a peptides also exert chemotactic influences on phagocytic monocytes and polymorphonuclear neutrophils. Coch-

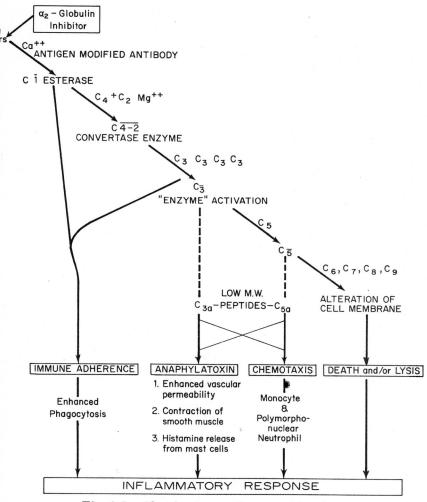

Fig. 4–1.—The classic complement pathway.

rane has shown that C3a and C5a activate mast cells, basophils and polymorphonuclear neutrophils effecting the release of contents from granules or lysosomes. Moreover, mast cells also exhibit membrane fusion under the influence of C3a and C5a.

COMPLEMENT-FIXATION TEST

The combination of sheep erythrocytes (SRBC's) with specific antibody in the presence of complement leads to lysis of the erythro-

Indicator System

SRBC's + Anti-SRBC's + Complement ⟶ Lysis of
                                                SRBC's
(Antigen)   (Antibody)   (C)

Complement Fixation Test

Positive Test   Test antigen + Serum containing antibody + C + Indicator = No Lysis
                                to test antigen   System   of SRBC's

Negative Test   Test antigen + Serum lacking antibody to + C + Indicator = Lysis of
                                test antigen   System   SRBC's

Fig. 4–2.—The complement-fixation test.

cyte through a puncture of the cell membrane and the subsequent loss
of hemoglobin into the fluid phase. This phenomenon is used as an
indicator system in the serologic testing of other antigen-antibody
reactions (Fig. 4-2). Classically, the complement-fixation reaction was
used in the serodiagnosis of syphilis (Wassermann test). In this test,
the patient's serum is mixed with an antigen that cross-reacts with
antigens of the syphilis spirochete, *Treponema pallidum.* The antigen
used is a lipoprotein (cardiolipin) prepared from bovine heart. A
carefully adjusted amount of guinea pig complement is added to the
antigen-serum mixture. If antibody is present in the serum being tested
and binds first antigen and then complement, inadequate amounts of
complement remain for reaction in the indicator system (SRBC's and
anti-SRBC's) as depicted in Figure 4-2. Complement-fixation tests are
currently used in the detection of antibody to viruses. In complement-
fixation reactions, Borsos and Rapp showed that a single molecule of
19S (IgM) antibody in combination with antigen at the cell surface is
adequate to bind one molecule of activated C1 whereas at least two or
more molecules of 7S antibody (IgG) in close proximity on the cell
surface are necessary to fix a molecule of the activated C1.

BIOLOGIC SIGNIFICANCE

The complement system or its components and products are intimately involved in several in vivo processes. *Beneficial effects* of
complement-fixation reactions undoubtedly play a role in host immunity to microbial parasites and involve the binding of complement
to antibodies attached to surface antigens of bacteria and viruses. The
microorganisms are subsequently either lysed (e.g., certain gram-
negative bacteria) or opsonized. With antibody-coated surfaces the
microorganisms are "sticky" and more readily ingested by host phago-

cytes; bound complement *contributes* to this "stickiness." In this manner, complement may facilitate the phagocytic ingestion of not only gram-negative and gram-positive bacteria but also of viruses.

Immunoconglutinin is a beneficial autoantibody directed against inner determinants of C3 (and possibly C4) which are exposed during in vivo fixations of complement. Consequently, immunoconglutinin enhances phagocytosis by reacting with its antigen (in C3) when C3 is bound in other antigen-antibody reactions and thereby contributing to the "stickiness" of the microorganism being opsonized.

As previously indicated, the activation of the complement system leads to a magnification of the host inflammatory response which is beneficial in clearing infectious microorganisms and necrotic host cells from the tissues. However, it may also be detrimental in certain autoimmune mechanisms such as immune complex deposition, a form of immunologic injury (see Chapter 9).

THE ALTERNATE COMPLEMENT PATHWAY

An alternate pathway for the activation of a portion of the complement system exists. It involves the components of the properdin system and appears to be the same as the C3 activator system. In the alternate complement pathway (Fig. 4-3) the C3 through C9 sequence of complement components is activated by endotoxins from gram-negative bacteria, zymosan (yeast cell wall polysaccharide) and inulin. Since the properdin system also spares the utilization of C1, C4 and C2

Fig. 4–3.—The alternate complement pathway.

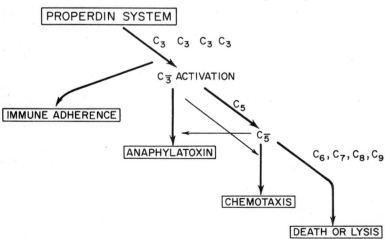

it does not require Ca^{++}. Properdin is comprised of normal serum factors and is involved in the neutralization of infectivity of some viruses. It is also bactericidal for certain gram-negative bacteria, e.g., Shigella species. It reacts with lipopolysaccharides (e.g., endotoxins), polysaccharides (e.g., zymosan and dextran) and with some immune complexes (antigen-antibody complexes) to form a complex which binds C3. Although not yet completely defined the properdin system consists of three serum factors: properdin, which is a protein distinct from any complement component or immunoglobulin; factor A, a hydrazine-sensitive serum protein; and factor B, a thermolabile pseudoglobulin which has recently been identified as a glycine-rich β-glycoprotein. Although the role of the properdin system in host resistance is well documented, its role in immunopathologic events is still being elucidated. Early in the discovery of the properdin system it was shown to be involved in the lysis of red blood cells of patients with paroxysmal nocturnal hemoglobinuria. A human patient has been described with an increased susceptibility to infection and decreased serum opsonizing, chemotactic and bactericidal function associated with a deficiency in factor B of the properdin system and C3. The alternate complement pathway and properdin system have also been indicated to function in initiating immunologic injury. The alternate pathway for C3 activation (involving the properdin system) may be of importance in host resistance to extracellular bacterial pathogens with carbohydrate capsules. Johnson and associates have observed that patients with deficiences in the alternate complement pathway who also have sickle-cell disorders are predisposed to infections by the gram-positive *D. pneumoniae* and the gram-negative *H. influenzae* (commonly found among the normal microflora of the upper respiratory tract). The alternate complement pathway and properdin system may function in the host defense of all humans against these particular bacterial pathogens prior to the formation of circulating antibody. The precise in vivo mechanisms by which serum properdin is reduced in pneumococcal pneumonia is not established. Coonrod suggests that serum properdin could be bound by the large quantities of pneumococcal polysaccharide (both soluble and bacteria-associated) which is produced during infection.

Recently, tick bite injury in rats was shown to be mediated by a complement-derived factor chemotactic for neutrophils. Tick salivary gland extracts exert no inherent chemotactic activity but are able to generate such action from human or canine serum. The serum factor acted upon by tick salivary gland extract was shown to be C5 and a cleavage product of C5 appeared to be the active chemotactic factor.

Complement depletion of C5 in the rats was achieved following injection of cobra venom. Markedly reduced inflammation and tissue necrosis at the site of the tick feeding lesion were seen in C5-depleted rats. Thus, the tissue injury following tick bite seems to be complement-mediated but *not* immunologically mediated.

INTERRELATION OF THREE HOST CASCADE SYSTEMS

Three host systems which appear to be interrelated seem most dramatically so in gram-negative endotoxin shock or disseminated intravascular coagulation (DIC). These three systems are the complement system, the blood clotting system and the kinin generation system. All of these are cascade type reactions in which the activation of one component leads to the sequential activation of others with the elaboration of vasoactive byproducts.

The Waterhouse-Friderichsen syndrome has classically been described as a sequel to meningococcemia (*Neisseria meningitidis* in the circulation). Although rare, this syndrome is manifested by thromboembolic lesions in the skin, joints, lungs and adrenals with adrenal hemorrhage. This condition in which acute adrenal insufficiency occurs *may* be a variation of disseminated intravascular coagulation (DIC).

DIC or endotoxin shock has been seen as a frequent complication of gram-negative bacteremias and sometimes as a complication in pneumococcal, rickettsial, fungal and mycobacterial infections. Endotoxins or endotoxin-like materials activate the complement, kinin and coagulation systems which in turn affect the microcirculation.

The following observations may be fragments of the dynamic events occurring in a patient undergoing endotoxin shock.

(1) Endotoxin is toxic to the vascular endothelium and the hepatic reticuloendothelial system.

(2) Since gram-negative bacteria are ubiquitous, antibodies to common microbial carbohydrate antigens, e.g., endotoxin carbohydrates, may frequently exist in individuals. (Bacterial endotoxins appear to be thymic-independent antigens and stimulate mainly IgM-type antibodies.) Some investigators feel that endotoxin shock is initiated by interactions of such antibody and endotoxin and complement.

(3) Both antigen-antibody complexes as well as endotoxin seem able to activate the kinin cascade. Kinins are a group of small polypeptides (9–11 amino acids) which are leukotactic and which can induce hypotension, increase vascular permeability, and affect the contractility of smooth muscle. Kallikrein is an enzyme which cleaves kinin

(bradykinin) from its precursor which is synthesized in the liver and liberated. Kinins are quickly inactivated by kinases and thus exhibit an extremely short half-life. The Hageman factor (coagulation factor XII) seems to be a necessary intermediate in the generation of kinins. The effects of kinins *may* contribute to the microcirculatory collapse in endotoxin shock since both patients and experimental animals with gram-negative bacteremia exhibit elevated levels of bradykinin and hypotension. McCabe observed that patients with fatal gram-negative bacteremia showed decreases in C3 levels in serum samples shortly after the onset of bacteremia. However, the inter-relationships of the kinins, coagulation and complement are still not clarified.

(4) Host cell necrosis induced by endotoxin may effect the release of lysosomal enzymes into the circulation. As a result, additional vascular injury (endothelial adherence, diapedesis of leukocytes, stasis of blood and petechial hemorrhage, degradation of vascular basement membrane, lysis of arterial elastic fibers, solubilization of collagen, release of histamine by mast cells, and increased vascular permeability) occurs. Thus, release of lysosomal enzymes contributes to the inflammatory response, the formation of clots, activation of the complement system, generation of kinins and fever.

Many investigators feel that DIC is really a Shwartzman-Sanarelli reaction. The Shwartzman-Sanarelli reaction has been a laboratory model for years. A local or systemic reaction can be induced in the rabbit based on the site selected for injection of either endotoxin or gram-negative bacteria containing endotoxin. If the site is intradermal (ID) a local reaction will ensue, while a generalized reaction may occur following intravenous (IV) injection. Approximately 8–24 hours after the priming injection, endotoxin or any colloidal substance (e.g., starch or agar) injected IV elicits either a local (at ID site) or a generalized (in IV-primed animal) reaction. The Shwartzman-Sanarelli reaction is evidenced by hemorrhagic necrosis and death in IV-primed animals. This is *not* an immunologic reaction since the time interval between the priming and eliciting doses is 24 hours or less and the reaction is not specific with respect to endotoxin. Endotoxin *must* be contained in the priming injection but need not even be present in the IV eliciting injection. Certain investigators feel that the initial dose of endotoxin induces vascular occlusion as a result of small inflammatory foci in the capillary beds. Then, when any colloidal material such as starch or agar or more endotoxin is injected into the circulation, extensive injury is triggered in the already occluded capillaries. This explanation is merely conjectural but logical.

The rabbit model is used as an experimental tool to study DIC. If the reticuloendothelial system of a rabbit is first blockaded by injection of carbon particles which are readily ingested by macrophages and vascular endothelial cells, then only one IV injection of endotoxin is needed to induce DIC. It is presumed that the blockage impairs clearance of endotoxin-induced fibrin aggregates by the reticuloendothelial system. Definitive proof that endotoxin actually produces all of these effects in the human patient is lacking.

COMPLEMENT DEFICIENCIES

Patients with hereditary angioneurotic edema lack serum alpha globulin inhibitor of C1. This defect is inherited as an autosomal dominant characteristic. The clinical entity is characterized "by recurrent, acute, circumscribed and transient subepithelial edema of the skin and mucosa of gastrointestinal and respiratory tracts" (Austen). The most severe aspect of this disease is acute laryngeal edema with death by asphyxiation. The mediator of the host damage is unknown although some investigators feel that it is a vasoactive peptide, possibly one of the kinins. Serum bradykinin levels are elevated in these patients during attacks.

A C2 deficiency has been documented in four persons homozygous for this deficit. None of the patients has shown any abnormal susceptibility to bacterial infections, although the sera of several of these patients in high dilutions exhibited impaired bactericidal reactions for *Salmonella typhosa.* (In vitro, gram-negative bacteria are killed in the presence of antibody and complement.) Subsequently low dilutions of their sera exhibited normal bactericidal activity. Later work found the alternate complement pathway intact in these patients. In an extensive review, Ruddy, Gigli and Austen cite that C1q deficiency appears to be associated with classic X-linked agammaglobulinemia and with the congenital lymphopenic form of severe combined immunodeficiency inherited in an autosomal recessive pattern. Afflicted children seem to suffer from chronic inflammatory problems and their sera do not exert normal bactericidal activity.

A familial C5 defect has been described in which a deficient opsonization (antibody and serum protein coating of bacteria which enhances phagocytic uptake) function was observed. The 18-month-old patient had experienced recurring infections by gram-negative bacteria.

A hypercatabolism of C3 has been noted in a patient with a lifelong history of infections. This patient also lacked both a C3 inactivator and properdin factor B. Müller-Eberhard described C1r, C2, C3 and C5 genetic deficiencies in man. The role of complement in host resistance and in immunologic injury is discussed in Chapters 8 and 9.

SUGGESTED READINGS

Alper, C. A.: Genetic Polymorphism of Complement Components as a Probe of Structure and Function, in Amos, B. (ed.): *Progress in Immunology I* (New York: Academic Press, 1971), p. 609.

Alper, C. A., *et al.*: Increased susceptibility to infection associated with abnormalities of C-mediated functions of the 3rd component of C (C3), N. Engl. J. Med. 282:349, 1970.

Austen, K. F.: Inborn errors of the complement system of man, N. Engl. J. Med. 276:1363, 1967.

Berenberg, J. L., Ward, P. A., and Sonenshine, D. E.: Tick-bite injury: Mediation by a complement-derived chemotactic factor, J. Immunol. 109:451, 1972.

Bokisch, V. A., *et al.*: The potential pathogenic role of complement in dengue hemorrhagic shock syndrome, N. Engl. J. Med. 289:996, 1973.

Borsos, T., Dournashkin, R. R., and Humphrey, J. H.: Lesions in erythrocyte membranes caused by immune hemolysis, Nature (London) 202:251, 1964.

Borsos, T., and Rapp, H. J.: Complement fixation on cell surfaces by 19S and 7S antibodies, Science 150:505, 1965.

Borsos, T., and Rapp, H. J.: Immune hemolysis: A simplified method for preparation of EAC'4 with guinea pig or with human complement, J. Immunol. 99:263, 1967.

Cochrane, C. G.: Initiating Events in Immune Complex Injury, in Amos, B. (ed.): *Progress in Immunology I* (New York: Academic Press, 1971), p. 143.

Coonrod, J. D.: Properdin levels in pneumonia (correspondence), N. Engl. J. Med. 288:1302, 1973.

Cooper, N. R.: Enzymes of the Complement System, in Amos, B. (ed.): *Progress in Immunology I* (New York: Academic Press, 1971), p. 567.

Gewurz, H.: The Immunologic Role of Complement, in Good, R. A., and Fisher, D. W. (eds.): *Immunobiology* (Stanford, Conn.: Sinauer Associates, Inc., Pub., 1971).

Gilbert, D. N., and Sanford, J. P.: Pathophysiology of Gram-negative Bacteremia, in Lauler, D. P. (ed.): *Gram-negative Sepsis* (Clifton, N. J.: Beecham Pharmaceuticals, Medcom, Inc., 1971).

Götze, O., and Müller-Eberhard, H. J.: The C3-activator system: An alternate pathway of complement activation, J. Exp. Med. 134:90, 1971.

Johnson, R. B., Newman, S. L., and Struth, A. G.: An abnormality of the alternate pathway of complement activation in sickle-cell disease, N. Engl. J. Med. 288:803, 1973.

Lepow, I. H.: Biologically Active Fragments of Complement, in Amos, B. (ed.): *Progress in Immunology I* (New York: Academic Press, 1971), p. 579.

Lepow, I. H., and Rosen, F. S.: Pathways to the complement systems, N. Engl. J. Med. 286:942, 1972.

Levin, J.: Endotoxin and endotoxemia (editorial), N. Engl. J. Med. 288:1297, 1973.

Mayer, M. M.: The complement system, Sci. Am. 229:54, 1973.

McCabe, W. R.: Serum complement levels in bacteremia due to gram-negative organisms, N. Engl. J. Med. 288:21, 1973.

Millar, K. G., and Mills, P.: $C_1 3$ and IgG levels in mothers and babies at delivery, Obstet. Gynecol. 39:527, 1972.

Müller-Eberhard, H. J.: Biochemistry of Complement, in Amos, B. (ed.): *Progress in Immunology I* (New York: Academic Press, 1971), p. 553.

Müller-Eberhard, H. J.: Complement and Human Disease, in Day, S. B., and Good, R. A. (eds.): *Membranes and Viruses in Immunopathology* (New York: Academic Press, 1972).

Naff, G. B.: Properdin—its biologic importance (editorial), N. Engl. J. Med. 287:716, 1972.

Pillemer, L., *et al.*: The properdin system and immunity. I. Demonstration and isolation of a new serum protein, properdin, and its role in immune phenomena, Science 120:279, 1954.

Polley, M. J.: Ultrastructural Studies of C1q and of Complement-Membrane Interactions, in Amos, B. (ed.): *Progress in Immunology I* (New York: Academic Press, 1971), p. 597.

Ratnoff, O. D.: The Interrelationship of Clotting and Immunologic Mechanisms, in Good, R. A., and Fisher, D. W. (ed.): *Immunobiology* (Stanford, Conn.: Sinauer Associates, Inc., Pub., 1971).

Rothfield, N., *et al.*: Glomerular and dermal deposition of properdin in systemic lupus erythematosus, N. Engl. J. Med. 287:681, 1972.

Ruddy, S., Gigli, I., and Austen, K. F.: The complement system of man, N. Engl. J. Med. (Part 1) 287:489; (Part 2) 287:545; (Part 3) 287:592; (Part 4) 287:642, 1972.

Stumacher, R. J., Kounat, M. J., and McCabe, W. R.: Limitations of the usefulness of the limulus assay for endotoxin, N. Engl. J. Med. 288:1261, 1973.

Ward, P. A.: Dengue, complement and shock (editorial), N. Engl. J. Med. 289:1034, 1973.

5 / Serology: Antigen-Antibody Interactions in Vitro

CHARACTERISTICS OF THE UNION OF ANTIBODY AND ANTIGEN

The combination of antigen and antibody is a specific yet reversible chemical reaction. The speed of the reversibility depends mainly upon the ability of each antibody Fab site to fit the three-dimensional conformation of its specific antigenic determinant. When the degree of fit is precise, binding of antibody to antigen is favored and the reversibility of the reaction is low; the antibody is then referred to as a high affinity antibody. When the degree of fit is poor, rapid dissociation of the antigen-antibody complex occurs; such antibody is referred to as low affinity antibody. Both antigen and antibody molecules are multivalent each having more than one reactive site per molecule and consequently combine in varying proportions. Except for the polymerized immunoglobulins such as IgM which has 10 antigen-binding sites, antibodies are usually restricted to two valences per molecule. In contrast, antigens are multivalent. Antigen valences may exceed 200 depending on the size and chemical complexity of the antigen, although they are more usually around 10 to 50 per molecule.

Particulate antigens such as red blood cells, leukocytes and bacteria react with their homologous antibodies to form agglutinated aggregates. Such reactions are termed *agglutination* reactions. Soluble antigens, such as serum proteins or bacterial polysaccharides (e.g., pneumococcal capsular substances) react with homologous antibodies to form precipitates. These reactions are termed *precipitin* reactions.

NATURE OF THE FORCES WHICH BIND ANTIGEN AND ANTIBODY

All antigen-antibody reactions occur in aqueous solution, in a charged ionic atmosphere, and between different sizes and shapes of molecules or particles. The combination occurs between a localized and very small part of the surface of the antibody molecule (Fab regions) and a correspondingly small part of the antigen. The tightness of this union depends upon how closely the surfaces can approach one another and upon the size of the areas involved; i.e., the antibody sites must fit the antigenic sites as exactly as possible for a "tight" fit. Although small variations in these sites can occur without spoiling the fit too badly, most variations will prevent binding. Thus, the combination of antigen and antibody shows a very high degree of specificity.

In biologic reactions such as enzyme-substrate and antigen-antibody interactions, stable covalent bonds are not formed between the two reactant molecules. If they were, dissociation of the complex would not occur and subsequent biologic function would be seriously impaired. (In certain enzyme-substrate interactions (covalent catalysis) an extremely unstable covalent enzyme-substrate complex forms and rapidly breaks down.)

The forces involved in the antigen-antibody binding depend partly upon the nature of the antigen. The extremely short range Van der Waals forces and hydrogen bonds are probably the most important.

(1) *Van der Waals forces* are effective binding forces at physiologic temperatures only when several atoms in a given molecule are bound to several atoms in another molecule. Then the energy of attraction is much greater than the dissociating tendency resulting from random thermal movements. In order for several atoms to interact effectively, the molecular fit must be precise. The strongest type of Van der Waals contact arises when a molecule contains a cavity exactly complementary in shape to a protruding group of another molecule, as in interactions of active sites of antigen-antibody and enzyme-substrate systems.

(2) *Hydrogen bonds* are weaker than covalent bonds, yet considerably stronger than Van der Waals bonds; i.e., a H-bond will hold two atoms closer together than the sum of their Van der Waals radii, but not as close together as a covalent bond will hold them.

Unlike Van der Waals bonds, hydrogen bonds are highly directional. In optimally strong hydrogen bonds, the hydrogen atom points directly at the acceptor atom. If it points indirectly, the bond energy is much less. Hydrogen bonds are also much more specific than Van der Waals bonds, since they demand the existence of molecules with complementary donor hydrogen and acceptor groups.

(3) *Electrostatic (Coulombic) forces* may also be involved in the binding of antigen and antibody if the antigenic determinant is ionically charged. In this instance the antibody will have a corresponding opposite ionic charge. The binding strength will be affected by the pH and ionic strength of the medium in which the antigen-antibody reaction takes place.

(4) Although *hydrophobic interactions* are not forces, they may also

contribute to the energy of binding. For example, an antigenic determinant which contains a phenyl group tends to surround itself with other nonpolar groups (those with low dielectric constants) and in so doing, is removed from the aqueous environment into the cleft of the Fab site of the antibody molecule. This accounts for the high energy of binding attributed to phenyl groups.

(5) In antigen-antibody interactions a *combination* of the total binding strengths of these forces contributes to the association of antigen and antibody molecules. These forces are usually maximal at physiologic conditions of pH and ionic strength. At pH values below 3 to 4 or above 10.5, they are often so much weaker that antigen-antibody complexes dissociate.

SPECIFICITY OF ANTIGEN-ANTIBODY INTERACTIONS

The combination of antigen and antibody is extraordinarily specific. Quite minor arrangements of the atoms in the antigenic determinant group will greatly reduce or even abolish its ability to combine with the original antibody. Antibodies, even against a given determinant made in a single individual, can vary markedly in their binding affinities.

Such variations are commonly expressed in terms of the *equilibrium constant, K,* derived from the classic expression for the Law of Mass Action. Hapten antigens and their antibodies best lend themselves to equilibrium dialysis studies.

$$K = \frac{[AbH]}{[Ab]\;[H]} \quad \frac{\text{association}}{\text{dissociation}} \qquad Ab + H \rightleftharpoons AbH$$

$[Ab]$ = antibody concentration in moles/liter at equilibrium
$[H]$ = hapten concentration in moles/liter at equilibrium
$[AbH]$ = concentration of antibody-hapten complex in moles/liter at equilibrium

K is expressed in liters/mole, and the higher its value, the greater the affinity of the antibody.

By determining the concentration of bound hapten in relation to the free hapten, the intrinsic association constant of the interaction of hapten and antibody can be determined from the equation:

$$K = \frac{[AbH]}{[Ab]\;[H]}$$

where $[Ab]$ = concentration of free antibody molecules, $[AbH]$ = concentration of antibody bound to hapten, and $[H]$ = concentration of free hapten.

K_0 is the average association constant, or the K value when one-half of the antibody sites are occupied with hapten. This is a more conveniently defined value, since antibody-hapten association constants are not uniform due to the many different antibody affinities in a given antiserum. In practice, values for K_0 may vary from 10^5 to 10^{12}, even for antibody against a single hapten group.

Antibody molecules of varying affinities occur during immunization. Usually, when an animal is first immunized against a hapten bound to carrier, the earliest antibodies formed have lower K_0 values than those formed later. Often a wide range of affinities occurs at all stages of immunization. When the immunogen is a complex protein, the earliest antibodies are usually not only of lower affinity, but are also more highly selective for that protein, in that they cross-react little, if at all, even with closely related antigens. As immunization is repeated or prolonged, the antibodies exhibit a higher affinity for antigen. Also, these antibodies cross-react with taxonomically related antigens but not with antigens which are wholly unrelated.

A plausible explanation for this broadening of specificity is as follows. The first antibodies formed are directed against only a few of the many determinant groups, i.e., the immunodominant groups. Also, certain evidence indicates that earliest antibody is directed against tertiary antigenic conformation. Thus, those groups most exposed in the tertiary antigenic structure may be those to which antibodies are first produced. The chance that these exposed groups are the same as those on related protein antigens is small. However, as immunization continues, antibodies are formed against a larger proportion of the determinant groups of the degraded antigen and the antiserum then contains a mixture of antibodies specific for a variety of different determinants, some of which are common to related antigen molecules.

IN VITRO REACTIONS

The unitarian theory of antibody reactivity was proposed by Zinsser. He considered it unreasonable to divide antibodies into agglutinating, precipitating or complement-fixing types, since it could be shown that, in some cases, the same antibody could perform all of these functions. However, in certain instances, a particular antibody may fail to accomplish a particular reaction. For example, certain antibodies fail to form visible precipitates with their homologous antigen and hence are termed nonprecipitating antibodies. In recent years, the heterogeneity of the antibody response to a given antigenic determinant affords an explanation for the failure of all antibodies to function serologically as Zinsser advocated. For example, there are four subclasses of human IgG and perhaps two subclasses of human IgM. Human IgA does not fix complement nor does one subclass of IgG.

In the union of antigen and antibody, there are essentially two stages: (1) primary interaction of association, and (2) secondary aggregation and cross-lattice formation of primary complexes leading to visible precipitation, agglutination, etc.

TITER

The *titer* is a term expressing the arbitrary approximation of antibody content in a serum sample. The antibody activity in serum is measured by adding a constant amount of test antigen to each of a row of tubes containing serially diluted antiserum. (For example, serum dilutions 1 in 2, 1 in 4, etc., or 1 in 10, 1 in 20, 1 in 40, etc.). The test antigen in an agglutination reaction is usually a certain amount of a calibrated suspension of either bacterial cells, erythrocytes, or other particulate antigens, while in a precipitation reaction, the test antigen usually is a solution containing protein or polysaccharide. After the mixtures of antigen and serum dilutions are prepared, they are incubated for a specified length of time and at a specified temperature (usually 37° C, but for the bacterial agglutinations, aggregations are enhanced by incubation at 45° to 55° C). After incubation, the tubes are observed to detect the endpoint of visible reactivity. For agglutination reactions, the last tube (highest dilution) of antiserum exhibiting aggregation of the cellular test antigen is considered the titer. In a complement-fixation titration, e.g., in a titration of rabbit anti-sheep-erythrocytes (hemolysin), the rabbit serum is diluted in a series of tubes, each of which contains a constant number of sheep erythrocytes and an adequate amount of complement. The titer, or endpoint, may be (1) the last tube showing complete hemolysis of the sheep erythrocytes or (2) for more accurate work, the tube showing lysis of approximately 50% of the red blood cells as determined photometrically. The last tube in the series which shows the desired effect may be considered to contain one arbitrary unit of antibody. The titer should be a measure of the number of antibody units per unit volume of the original serum. Thus, if the last tube showing a reaction contains a 1-ml volume, and the serum in *this tube* is diluted 1 in 640, the titer of the serum is 640 units per milliliter of serum.

APPLICATIONS OF SEROLOGIC TESTS IN DIAGNOSIS

CHANGING TITER.—The presence of an elevated titer of antibodies to a particular microorganism indicates *only* that infection or vaccination has occurred at some time in the past. In order to establish that an acute illness is due to a given microorganism, it is desirable to show a *change* in titer to that agent during the illness (i.e., the absence of detectable antibodies during the first week, their appearance, and progressive increase in titer during the second and subsequent weeks and, perhaps, their eventual decline). For practical purposes, a *pair* of serum samples are compared—one from the acute phase and one from the convalescent phase of the illness. If only a single serum sample is available late in the illness, a high titer for the microbial agent is sometimes accepted as provisional diagnostic evidence. Under these circumstances, it is necessary to be certain that the high titer is not the result of prior vaccination. In order to prove that an isolated microorganism is the etiologic agent of the illness, it is desirable to use the isolate as test antigen in the serologic tests.

IDENTIFICATION OF ETIOLOGIC AGENT.—Even when no likely agent has been isolated, a provisional etiologic diagnosis can be made by testing the serum with various microbial antigens. The antigen which gives the highest titer is assumed to be from the etiologic agent. However, this procedure may be misleading, since other antigens not tested may have reacted in higher titer with the serum tested. Also, some curious cross-reactions between very different microorganisms may tend to mislead; e.g., persons with rickettsial infections form antibodies in high titer to certain *Proteus X* strains, while some persons with *Mycoplasma pneumoniae* infections form cold hemagglutinins as well as agglutinins to an alpha hemolytic streptococcus known as strep-MG.

TIME COURSE.—In the course of a given infectious disease, the appearance and persistence of antibodies to the etiologic agent follow a different time course when measured with different antigenic preparations and different serologic tests. For example, in brucellosis, agglutination titers appear early in infection and persist at low levels for years afterward, whereas precipitin levels appear later and disappear much sooner. In many rickettsial and viral diseases, the antibody titers measured by complement fixation appear later and subside sooner than those measured by neutralization.

In determining a titer of antibody activity in a serum sample, certain considerations must be recognized. Agglutinin (antibody which agglutinates) titers obtained with different bacteria are not comparable because the number and distribution of antigenic determinant groups on the bacterial cell surface can influence titer to a marked degree. Thus, a given microorganism is obviously an assembled mosaic of

TABLE 5.1—SENSITIVITY OF VARIOUS METHODS OF DETECTING ANTIBODIES*

METHOD	μG OF ANTIBODY N/ML†
Autoradiography	0.0002
Qualitative ring precipitation test	3–5
Precipitation in gels	5–10
Quantitative micro-Kjeldahl nitrogen	10
Colorimetry (Folin and Ciocalteu)	4
Bacterial agglutination	0.01
Bactericidal (with optimum complement)	
turbimetric	0.001
viable count	0.00001
Passive hemagglutination	0.003–0.006
Hemolysis (lytic antibody + complement)	0.001–0.03
Complement fixation	0.05–0.1
Flocculation test (syphilis)	0.2–0.5
Toxin neutralization—diphtheria antitoxin in rabbit skins	0.01

	TOTAL ANTIBODY REQUIRED (μg N)
Passive anaphylaxis in whole guinea pig	30
Passive anaphylaxis with guinea pig uterine muscle	0.01
Passive cutaneous anaphylaxis guinea pig skin	0.003
Skin transfer (Prausnitz-Küstner) in human	0.01

*Modified from Humphrey, J. H., and White, R. G., 1970.
†Multiply by 6.25 to obtain antibody protein.

many antigens which differ in amount, immunogenicity and stability in the animal host.

There are structural and functional differences in the antibodies specific for a given antigenic determinant, and different types of antibodies are formed at different stages in the immune response.

The various serologic methods differ in their sensitivity (Table 5-1).

IMMUNE PRECIPITATION REACTIONS

In precipitation reactions the test antigens are soluble molecules such as proteins or polysaccharides. The antibody which reacts with soluble antigens is referred to as a *precipitin.* Under optimal conditions, the reaction occurs rapidly and may be complete within a few seconds. The visible precipitate contains both antigen and antibody as components as well as other serum components such as complement, if present in the reacting system. Complement is *not* necessary for the union of antigen and antibody. Most antibody molecules are bivalent and, even though soluble, the precipitating antigens are multivalent. These reactants combine and eventually form three-dimensional structures or lattices which precipitate out of solution.

In titrations for precipitating antibody activity, those tubes in which a visible turbidity is first observed usually contain the zone of equivalence or optimal proportions (Fig. 5-1,B). In these reactions, all of the valences of the antibody and antigen molecules have interacted and no free antigen or antibody can be detected in the supernatant fluid (Fig. 5-1,D). Also, the antibody content of that serum can be calculated by examining the precipitate. In mixtures of antigen and antibody in which the multivalent antigen is present in excess amounts, little or no precipitate is seen (Fig. 5-1,C). This is because the antibody molecules present in limited numbers react in solution with antigen to form soluble complexes. Lattice formation cannot occur. When the situation is reversed and antibody molecules are in excess, lattice formation does occur and insoluble complexes are seen as visible precipitates. Reactions in this zone of antibody excess afford a means for estimating the valence of the particular test antigen being utilized (e.g., in Fig. 5-1,A). On occasion, in regions of extreme antibody excess, the antigen-antibody complexes which form are too small to be visible. This situation occurs more readily when the precipitating antigen is of low valence and in the sera of certain species (such as horse and human).

VARIATIONS OF THE PRECIPITIN TEST

(1) A *precipitin ring* test is performed in tubes of small diameter or even in capillary tubes where antigen solution is carefully layered

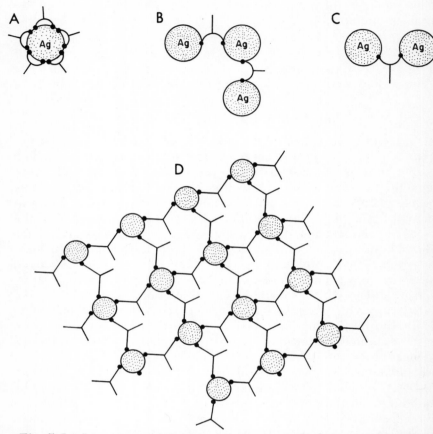

Fig. 5-1.—Immune precipitation. A, extreme antibody excess. B, optimal proportions of antigen and antibody. C, antigen excess. D, lattice formation = visible precipitation.

either over or under the serum containing antibody. At the interface, a region of optimal proportions is reached and a visible precipitate forms. This method yields visible precipitates in a short time when the serum being used contains high titers of precipitating antibody.

(2) The *Quellung reaction* is shown diagrammatically in Figure 5-2. In this reaction, the pneumococcus *(D. pneumoniae)* which contains type-specific polysaccharide capsules is reacted with antiserum (serum containing antibodies). In the example shown the encapsulated pneumococcus possesses type I capsule. In the presence of specific antibody (anti-type I polysaccharide) an immune precipitation reaction

occurs and the capsule can be seen microscopically to swell. When antibody against another capsular type of pneumococcus, e.g., anti-type III, is applied to the type I pneumococcus, no precipitate forms and no capsular swelling is seen.

(3) In clinical immunology, the *Ouchterlony double diffusion* method of immune precipitation in agar gel (agarose) is used. This method involves the placement of antigen and antibody preparations in separate wells cut in the agar. The soluble reactants (antigen and serum containing antibody) diffuse through the gel and a line or lines of precipitation occur in the areas where they meet in optimal proportions. By this method several distinct antigenic moieties contained in the test antigen will form separate and identifiable lines of precipitate with specific antisera. Moreover, antigenic relatedness is readily shown by this technic. As shown in Figure 5-3, when a serum sample containing both anti-X and anti-Y is placed in a well in the agar and purified preparations of X and Y antigens are placed in separate wells, two distinct lines of precipitate form which bisect one another. This indicates that antigens X and Y are not identical. Identity of antigens by this method is shown in the diagram marked *Identity.* In this situation the antiserum contains anti-M and anti-N and both test antigen wells contain antigens M and N. Consequently, the lines

Fig. 5–2.—Diagrammatic representation of a Quellung reaction.

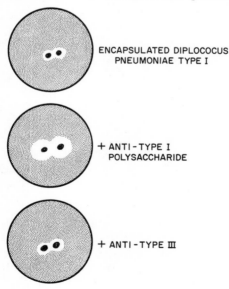

ENCAPSULATED DIPLOCOCUS
PNEUMONIAE TYPE I

+ ANTI-TYPE I
POLYSACCHARIDE

+ ANTI-TYPE III

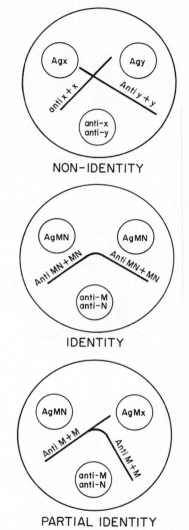

NON-IDENTITY

IDENTITY

PARTIAL IDENTITY

Fig. 5–3.—Ouchterlony double diffusion reactions.

formed in each system are confluent and form an arc at their inter-
section.

When two antigen preparations contain common antigenic groups as
well as distinct antigenic moieties, the precipitation lines which form
are characteristic of this partial identity as shown in the diagram

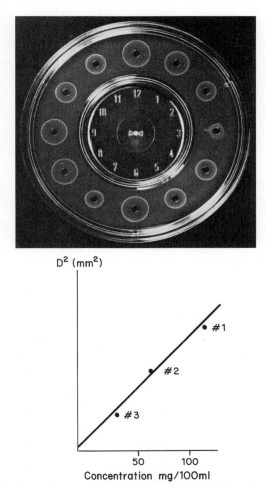

Fig. 5-4.—Radial immunodiffusion and estimation of serum C3 content. *Wells 1, 2, and 3* in the gel diffusion plate (*top*) contain three different concentrations of a serum protein standard. The diameters of the precipitate formed in wells 5-12 may be measured, squared and the serum complement (C3) levels of each sample read from the *graph (bottom)*.

labeled *Partial identity*. In this example lines of identity form between the M antigens and the anti-M while a precipitin spur forms over this arc between the distinct antigen N and its antibody.

(4) A variation of this method which affords quantitation of an antigen is the method of *radial immunodiffusion*. In this sensitive

procedure specific antibody is incorporated in the agar gel and antigen is placed in wells cut in the agar. A quantitation of C3 (B_1C globulin) serum levels is shown in Figure 5-4. The area of precipitate formed around each antigen well is measured. Higher concentrations of antigen diffuse farther from the well before the concentration is diminished to the level reacting in optimal proportions. The level of serum complement for each sample is read from a standard curve determined simultaneously with the test. Calibrated amounts of C3 are used to establish the standard curve. This method is used routinely not only to quantitate serum levels of complement, but also to determine immunoglobulin levels, particularly in hypogammaglobulinemic or myeloma patients. It is also used to determine transferrin and C-reactive protein levels and the levels of many other plasma proteins.

(5)*Haptens* are used to inhibit specific precipitation reactions. By allowing the hapten the opportunity to react first with the specific antibody, the complete antigen (hapten conjugated to carrier protein) is unable to find enough Fab portions of antibody free to form a visible precipitate. This situation is somewhat analogous to antigen excess.

(6) In *immunoelectrophoresis* as shown in Figure 5-5 an antigen sample (human serum) is first subjected to electrophoresis in agar gel mounted on glass slides. Subsequently, antiserum containing antibody is placed in a trough which has been cut in the agar on each slide. The slides are incubated in a moist atmosphere to allow precipitation lines to form. In Figure 5-5 a normal human serum sample and a serum sample from a patient with an IgG myeloma are reacted with goat anti-human serum after electrophoresis. Note the heavy band of precipitate formed between the IgG of the myeloma patient and the antiserum trough.

Fig. 5–5.—Immunoelectrophoresis of human sera: IgG myeloma protein compared with normal serum IgG. *Top*, immunoelectrophoretic pattern of human IgG myeloma serum; note the extensive amount of precipitate in the arc (M) on the left in the presence of anti-human serum (AHS). *Bottom*, immunoelectrophoretic pattern of normal human serum (N) in the presence of anti-human serum.

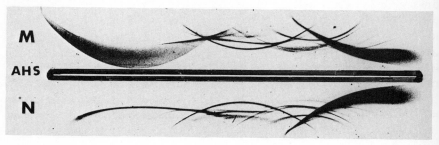

(7) Combining the technics of electrophoresis in agar gel with immunoprecipitation has yielded several other useful applications. *Counter immunoelectrophoresis* cannot be used with any antigen except those that migrate rapidly toward the anode at pH 8.2 to 8.6, e.g., hepatitis B antigen of human serum (HBAg). The test serum containing antibody is placed in a well closer to the anode while the test antigen (e.g., HBAg) is placed in the agar gel in a well near the serum well but on the cathodal side. Since the antibody-containing gamma globulin serum fraction migrates toward the cathode at pH 8.2 to 8.6 and the HBAg migrates as an alpha$_2$ globulin toward the anode in electrophoresis, application of electric current actually speeds up the migration of the antigen and antibody through the gel to form an immunoprecipitation line.

(8) *Electroimmunodiffusion* may be used to quantitate proteins in low concentrations, e.g., those in cerebrospinal fluid. This assay is a variation of radial immunodiffusion in that a monospecific antiserum is incorporated in the agar. Multiple wells containing various test antigens are placed toward the cathodal side of the slide. Current is applied for a specified time and the height of the resulting precipitin arc (rocket) forming for each sample is proportional to the concentration of that substance. This rapid method is useful for quantitating cerebrospinal fluid proteins including immunoglobulin.

(9) *Quantitative immunoelectrophoresis* is not a clinical but a research tool. It employs high voltage (300 V) electrophoresis and involves active electroimmunodiffusion in one direction followed by immunoelectrophoresis in a perpendicular plane in agar gel.

(10) *Radioimmunoassay technics* are extremely valuable tools in determining serum body fluid levels of IgE, carcinoembryonic antigen (CEA) and hormones by measuring the binding of radiolabeled antigen to a specific amount of antibody. In the test, the antigen sample is allowed first to react with a fixed amount of antibody and then the radiolabeled antigen-antibody binding is determined. In this manner, the serum or body fluid component being assayed competes with the labeled antigen for the antibody. Thus, the partial inhibition of binding by the labeled antigen may be determined.

(11) In the *fluorescent antibody technic* labeled antibody is allowed to react with antigen, which is usually part of a cell. This technic is useful clinically in the determination of anti-nuclear antibody (ANA) in sera of patients with lupus erythematosus and in identifying microorganisms from clinical specimens.

The *direct procedure* involves the utilization of specific antibody labeled with a fluorescent dye (usually fluorescein isothiocyanate or lissamine rhodamine B). After the labeled antiserum is reacted with the antigen preparations, the preparations are washed and then viewed under a (fluorescent) microscope employing an ultraviolet light source The areas of specific antigen-antibody interaction will emit a brigh apple-green fluorescence when fluorescein isothiocyanate is used.

The *indirect procedure* is more practical for routine laboratory use but requires technical skill and carefully prepared controls. In thi method, unlabeled antibody is reacted with the test antigen (eithe frozen tissue or bacteria) and the specimen is then washed with saline Next, labeled antiserum directed against the antibody (e.g., goa anti-human globulin) is added to the slide and the specimen is viewed as before. This particular procedure is used routinely in the ANA tes and in the diagnosis of syphilis.

THE AGGLUTINATION REACTION

In the agglutination reaction, cells or other particulate substance are used as test antigens. A *direct hemagglutination* reaction consists o adding erythrocytes which contain a given antigen to a serum contain ing antibody. This procedure is used mainly as a hematologic pro cedure in blood banks in the typing of erythrocyte antigens. For example, red cells containing blood group A antigen will agglutinate ir anti-A but not anti-B sera.

Hemagglutination-inhibition reactions have been used in the pas with Rh_0 blocking antibody. The human anti-Rh_0(D) of the IgG class does not appear either to bind complement or to agglutinate directly human erythrocytes bearing Rh_0(D) antigen IgG. Anti-human red cel antibody of the human IgG class does not form visible agglutinate directly, although it does bind to erythrocyte antigens. When Rh_0(D red cells are first reacted with this IgG type antibody, the Rh_0(D) active sites are blocked from forming visible agglutination with the IgM class of anti-Rh_0(D).

The *passive hemagglutination* test is a useful and very sensitive serologic procedure. In this procedure red cells are passively used as "carrier" surfaces. Antigens such as carbohydrates may be directly coated onto erythrocytes, and protein or nucleoprotein antigens can be coupled (via bis-diazotized benzidine, chromium chloride, or glutaral dehyde) to red cell surfaces. Consequently, the red cell to which the test antigen is attached can then be used to detect specific antibodies to that test antigen in the easy-to-visualize agglutination reaction.

This principle has been utilized in the detection of rheumatoid factor (an IgM antibody directed against denatured gamma chains of IgG) in human serum. Particulate vehicles other than red cells, such as latex or bentonite (clay) particles, may be used to carry the antigen. The most common procedure for detecting rheumatoid factor in human serum utilizes latex particles coated with denatured H chains of human IgG.

In syphilis serology the VDRL test is used as a screening test. This is a flocculation test in which a patient's serum is reacted with a particulate cardiolipin material. If aggregation occurs, the test is positive.

The Coombs' test is of great diagnostic value in the verification of autoimmune hemolytic anemias. Normally, washed human erythrocytes contain no immunoglobulins when placed in anti-human globulin serum. But the red cells of patients with autoimmune hemolytic anemia, even after careful washings in chilled saline, will usually be agglutinated after incubation for 30 minutes at 37° C in anti-human globulin serum (Coombs' serum). The erythrocytes of human neonates with erythroblastosis fetalis or of adults with acquired autoimmune hemolytic disease will be "Coombs positive" in this test.

In the *indirect Coombs' test*, serum which contains antibody to an erythrocyte antigen (e.g., the maternal serum of an infant with erythroblastosis fetalis contains anti-Rh_o[D]) is used to passively coat red cells containing that antigen. (Remember that human IgG anti-red cell antibody reacts with but does not form visible agglutinates with red cells bearing that antigen.) The cells so treated are washed in chilled saline and Coombs' serum is added to them as described for the direct Coombs' test. Such treated cells will agglutinate.

Bacteria are agglutinated by antibody. The flagellated enteric bacilli form a loose, "fluffy" agglutination in antiflagellar serum while those bacilli reacting with anti-O serum form a tighter agglutination. Also, the motile spirochetes such as Leptospira species are immobilized in their agglutination by antibody. It is of interest to note that of all the bacteria, only with the leptospira and mycoplasma is the multiplication inhibited by antibody directed against surface antigens.

In virology, certain groups of viruses will adsorb to the erythrocytes of certain species giving a characteristic "shieldlike" agglutination pattern. The red cells to which virus is adsorbed settle to the bottom of the tube in an agglutinated pattern. If, however, the virus is first mixed with specific antibody and the susceptible red cells are then added to this mixture, the red cells are not hemagglutinated but settle as do control cells in a compact button- or donut-shaped mass. This procedure is called an *hemagglutination-inhibition test* and is used routinely in the serodiagnosis of certain viral infections. In fact, this is the *best* procedure to determine whether one has ever had a mumps infection.

For some reason, most people after mumps infection retain a detectable titer of hemagglutination-inhibition antibody thereafter.

COMPLEMENT FIXATION

The principle of this procedure is described in Chapter 4. The Wassermann test, used for years in the serodiagnosis of syphilis, is a complement-fixation test. Currently, complement-fixation tests are more widely used in virology laboratories and in the serodiagnosis of viral infections.

TISSUE TYPING

An early procedure used in the detection of histocompatibility HL-A antigens was *leukoagglutination* in which antiserum agglutinates blood leukocytes. Antisera used in HL-A typing are usually obtained from multiparous females and from individuals who have received multiple transfusions of whole blood. Over 95% of the possible HL-A alleles in both the LA and Four series can be recognized serologically. To date, the LA locus of the human species is responsible for more than 10 allelomorphic antigens while the Four locus seems to control more than 20 such antigens. Recall that the cells of each individual display four HL-A antigenic specificities (two LA and two Four). Each parent contributes one LA and one Four specificity to a given individual. When all four HL-A specificities are detected serologically, this recognition is termed "full house."

In the typing of recipients and donors for a possible tissue transplantation, the ABO erythrocyte antigens are determined by direct hemagglutination methods with commercial typing serum. HL-A antigens are present in most tissues. Most test procedures used in tissue typing use peripheral blood leukocytes as the source of HL-A antigens. However, platelets may be used for HL-A typing. A quantitative complement-fixation test may be used in which the free complement not bound by platelet antigens and anti-HL-A lyses antibody-sensitized red cells. The amount of hemoglobin released by the sheep red cells is quantitated spectrophotometrically. However, prior to use in HL-A testing, the platelets must stand for 2 to 3 days at 4° C for activation of the HL-A antigens. The HL-A antigens in the platelets of freshly drawn blood are not active. Once prepared, the platelet HL-A antigens are stable in saline for 10–12 months and can be stored frozen in liquid nitrogen.

The previously mentioned leukoagglutination test is the least sensitive and most specific assay. *Cytotoxicity* testing is more sensitive and involves an incubation of the test cells with a standard antiserum and complement. The cells are then scored for viability. Any cell which has been killed is presumed to contain the HL-A antigen specificity of the antibody in the test serum. The test cells may be stained with a vital dye, e.g., trypan blue. Dead cells take up the dye while living cells do not. Or, the test cells may be preincubated with radiolabeled chromium prior to cytotoxicity testing. Using this method, the amount of labeled chromium released when the cells are killed (by the action of antibody and complement) can be measured. The *microabsorption technic* is a variation of cytotoxicity testing. A tissue homogenate of the donor is used in the presence of complement to absorb each test antiserum. The absorbed antiserum is then exposed to lymphocytes (test cells) from an individual known to carry the HL-A specificity of the unabsorbed antiserum. The test cells are then stained with trypan blue and viability determined microscopically. If the test cells take up the dye, antibody was not absorbed by the donor tissue extract and that HL-A specificity is not present in the donor. The mixed lymphocyte blastogenic reaction measuring the MLC (mixed lymphocyte culture) locus was originally thought to measure only HL-A specificities. Apparently, it does not. This test and its relation to HL-A typing is discussed in Chapter 11.

IMMUNOCYTOADHERENCE: MIXED CELL AGGLUTINATION REACTIONS OR ROSETTE TESTS

For the sake of simplicity in discussion, this reaction will be referred to as the rosette test. In essence, specific T cells or specific immunoglobulin receptors on B cells or antibody attached by its Fc region (*cytophilic antibody*) to macrophage membranes can bind antigens displayed on a cell surface. Complement receptors for C3 on B cells and macrophages can be demonstrated by rosette formation. The result visualized microscopically is the formation of a rosette, i.e., a central mononuclear cell surrounded by cells containing antigen. The rosette test has been used to visualize bacterial surface antigens attached to macrophages via cytophilic antibody and sheep red blood cell antigens attached to B cells and T cells (see Chapter 7).

A variation of this test involves the binding of major blood group antigens of human erythrocytes via specific anti-blood group antibody bridges to human tissues displaying the same blood group antigenicity. Immunocytoadherence is viewed microscopically as red cell adherence to cells contained in tissue sections.

SUGGESTED READINGS

Davis, B. D., Dulbecco, R., Eisen, H. N., Ginsberg, H. S., Wood, W. B., Jr., and McCarthy, M.: *Microbiology* (2nd ed.; Hagerstown, Md.: Harper & Row, Publishers, 1973).

Haaf, E. (ed.): *Lab Synopsis,* Diagnostic Reagents Bulletin (Woodbury, N. Y.: Behring Diagnostics, Inc., 1969).

Humphrey, J. A., and White, R. G. (eds.): *Immunology for Students of Medicine* (3rd ed.; Philadelphia: F. A. Davis Co., 1970).

Kabat, E. A., and Mayer, M. M.: *Experimental Immunochemistry,* 2nd ed. (Springfield, Ill.: Charles C Thomas, 1961).

Lehninger, A. L.: *Biochemistry* (New York: Worth Publishers, Inc., 1970).

Watson, J. D.: *Molecular Biology of the Gene* (2nd ed.; New York: W. A. Benjamin, Inc., 1970).

Weir, D. M. (ed.): *Handbook of Experimental Immunology* (Philadelphia: F. A. Davis, Co., 1967).

6 / Cell-Mediated Immunity

The T lymphocyte system is responsible for cell-mediated immune phenomena. Cell-mediated immunity appears to be independent of both B lymphocytes and antibody. The prototypes of cell-mediated immune host reactions are delayed hypersensitivity (DH), allograft rejection and graft-versus-host (GVH) reactions.

Delayed hypersensitivity to microbial antigens has long been recognized and has been classically referred to as the "allergy of infection." The significance of these responses was, until recently, not well understood. The classic delayed allergies studied were the tuberculin skin test sensitivity and poison ivy (a contact dermatitis).

Certain antigens appear to stimulate T cells to proliferate. As a consequence, an increase in the number of specific antigen-reactive T cells occurs in a sensitized individual. Responsiveness of these cells can be detected upon skin testing with antigen.

The onset of visible cell-mediated skin reactivity requires time (48–96 hours) after antigen injection and hence the terms delayed hypersensitivity or delayed allergy are used to differentiate these skin test responses from those which appear immediately. IgE-mediated responses appear within minutes of antigen injection. Arthus type reactions (IgM, IgG and complement-mediated) first appear 4–6 hours after antigen injection and may last as long as 36 hours.

Histologically the delayed type hypersensitive skin response is characterized by the infiltration of mononuclear cells (macrophages and lymphocytes). The other types of skin reactions are characterized more as local inflammatory responses. Grossly, the positive delayed skin responses are indurated (hard), and if an intensive reaction has occurred, the reaction may exhibit a necrotic center. The time of appearance of a delayed skin test response varies. In general, it first appears within 24–48 hours after antigen injection and is maximum at 72–96 hours. The response may remain visible for *more* than 7 days.

A Jones-Mote type skin response may be confused with a delayed hypersensitive skin reaction. It generally appears sooner (within 24 hours) and fades earlier (by 4 days). The curious response may be the result of a partially suppressed T cell response to antigen. However, a the Jones-Mote reaction is waning, plasma cells may be seen at the site indicating that the effector lymphocytes reactive with skin-test antigen may have been B cells. Jones-Mote reactions were first described early in the course of the antibody response to protein antigens such a diphtheria or tetanus toxoids, e.g., at 6 days following immunization With tuberculin testing of humans, care must be taken in interpreting skin test reactions, for all types of skin responses may be seen on occasion.

The sequence of events leading to a delayed type hypersensitive skin response is probably as follows. T cells present or coming into the site of antigen injection react with antigen and release a variety of soluble effector molecules called lymphokines. The lymphokines are biochemical mediators and are probably responsible for effecting the so-called cell-mediated immune response seen in tissues. At least 13 different effector responses have been seen, but whether 13 separate molecules exist is unknown.

LYMPHOKINES

Lymphokines are the effector molecules elaborated by specific antigen-reactive T lymphocytes in the presence of antigen. To date, most studies of lymphokine activities have been performed in in vitro systems; migration inhibitory factor (MIF) is the best characterized of these substances. The release of MIF from T lymphocytes need not require proliferation of the T cell in the guinea pig but may in the human. MIF appears to trap macrophages, inhibiting their migration. In the guinea pig, MIF apparently is a glycoprotein since it is sensitive to the action of both chymotrypsin and neuraminidase. However, human MIF appears to be mainly protein since it is sensitive to the action of chymotrypsin but resistant to neuraminidase. MIF may possibly be the same as *macrophage aggregating factor* which some investigators have assayed as a lymphokine. At present, it is uncertain whether MIF also contains *macrophage activating factor*. Macrophage activating factor activates macrophages metabolically to exhibit heightened microbicidal capacity. Certain studies have indicated that MIF and macrophage activating factor are the same substance while other studies have not.

MIF is distinct from *blastogenic factor*, a proteinaceous lymphokine which induces lymphoid cells to proliferate. The effects of blastogenic factor may be determined by enumerating the number of lymphoid cells undergoing blast transformation after culture in the presence of antigen. Blastogenesis is more sensitively assayed by measuring the uptake of a labeled precursor molecule (such as H^3-thymidine) which is added to lymphocytes cultured in the presence of antigen for several days. Some investigators have even reported that a *blastogenic inhibitor factor* may be released as a lymphokine. The circumstances under which this occurs are unclear.

Plant mitogens such as phytohemagglutinin (PHA) and concanavalin A can stimulate T lymphocytes to a blastogenic response. They also effect a release of MIF and skin *reactive factors* from nonimmune T cells much as does antigen when exposed to immune T cells. Since antigen stimulates release of lymphokines from antigen-specific T cells, the nonspecific plant mitogens may induce all available T cells in culture to produce and release lymphokines. Apparently, concanavalin A does exert this effect. In one study, concanavalin A-treated lymphoid cells showed 10 times greater MIF activity than did immune lymphoid cells incubated with optimal amounts of specific antigen.

Lymphotoxin or *lymphocytotoxin* is a protein substance liberated from T lymphocytes stimulated with antigen or concanavalin A. The lymphotoxin is more cytotoxic for other host cells than for lymphocytes. Originally, this toxic lymphokine was described as being released from T cells sensitive to tuberculin (purified protein derivative, PPD). Its contribution to tissue necrosis in patients with tuberculosis is suggested; the onset of caseous necrosis correlates with the earliest manifestations of positive tuberculin skin tests. The necrotic effects of the so-called "killer" lymphocytes described in the killing of tumor cells may also be the result of elaboration of lymphotoxin. In the in vitro demonstration of "killer" lymphocytes, immune lymphocytes are seen situated next to the antigen-laden target cell with direct contact between lymphocyte and target cell membranes. Many investigators have felt that the tumoricidal activity of immune lymphoid cells is the result of a different killing mechanism than that effected by lymphotoxin. However, this need not be so. Lymphotoxin may be elaborated by the "killer" T cell directly into or at the membrane of the abutting target cell.

A *proliferative inhibitory* factor (PIF) is produced by either immune or PHA-stimulated lymphocytes following direct contact with target cells (tumor cells). The tumor cells are inhibited from growth but not killed by PIF. The effects of PIF are reversible if lymphocytes are removed; however, the tumor cells require several days to reinitiate visible growth. No cytotoxic factors were found in these culture supernatant fluids, which suggests that inhibition of tumor cell growth resulted from contact with the immune lymphocyte membrane. PIF is a macromolecule produced by stimulated human lymphocytes and not by unstimulated lymphocytes.

Chemotactic factors for macrophages and polymorphonuclear neutrophils (PMN's), interferon and transfer factors are also considered as lymphokines.

T CELL SYSTEM

The T cell system is a complex, and, in many ways, still an ill-defined system of lymphocytes. T cells have antigen-specific receptors which, in contrast to receptors of B cells, are *not* immunoglobulin molecules. Functional subclasses of T cells have been described based upon the presence or absence of a cell-surface marker sensitivity to x-irradiation and/or corticosteroids. The theta antigen is a marker for mouse T cells. The "primitive" T cell present in yolk sac, fetal liver and bone marrow is considered a *prethymic* cell and does not exhibit theta antigen. This cell is not immunologically competent. In mice, it is radiosensitive and normally migrates to thymus and bone marrow. Within the thymus a series of essential yet unknown events occurs. Even though most thymus lymphocytes are unable to respond to antigen (immunologically incompetent), Raff indicates that about 2–5% of thymus cells are immunocompetent and located in the thymus medulla.

At least five types of T cells are considered post-thymic cells and are designated as T_1, T_2, T_3, T_4 and T_5. T_1 cells are not yet immunocompetent, bear theta antigen and are sensitive to humoral products of the thymus which induce their differentiation to T_2 cells. T_1 cells are present in fetal liver, neonatal spleen and in peripheral lymphoid tissues. T_2 cells also bear theta antigen and are the long-lived immunocompetent recirculating cells responsible for immunosurveillance (see Chapter 7). They are found in the blood, lymph and thymus-dependent areas of peripheral lymphoid tissues. T_3 cells, present in the peripheral lymphoid tissues, are selectively mobilized via the blood to sites of inflammatory exudates. T_3 cells do not recirculate from blood to lymph and back as do T_2 cells. T_3 cells bear specific antigen receptors and produce lymphokines. T cell immunologic memory may reside in the radioresistant, theta-positive T_2 and T_4 cells. T_4 cells reside in the spleen, lymph nodes and bone marrow and are capable of inducing the radiosensitive nonspecific (prethymic) bone marrow cells to accomplish cell-mediated immune reactions. The T_5 cells are situated in locales where they may well be the T cells which exert "helper" function to B cells in the T cell-dependent antibody responses. T_5 cells are found in the thymus-dependent areas of spleen and lymph nodes as well as in the blood and thymic cortex. In mice, T_5 cells are sensitive to both steroids and x-irradiation. In comparison to T_2 cells, they are short-lived (Good considers them short-lived memory cells).

ASSAYS OF T CELL FUNCTION

In order to assay T cell function in humans, a variety of methods now exist. To determine T cell responsiveness of the peripheral white blood cells, the in vitro transformation (blastogenic response) to the mitogen phytohemagglutinin (PHA) can be readily measured and quantitated. The capacity to form new delayed type hypersensitivity reactions may be determined by attempting to sensitize the patient via the skin with antigens that are not commonly found in the human environment. Antigens used in this manner are 2,4-dinitrochlorobenzene (DNCB), which is painted on the skin in an alcoholic solution to establish contact sensitivity, or the more potent antigen keyhole limpet hemocyanin (KLH), which may be injected intradermally. After sensitization (usually 2–3 weeks) the patient is skin tested with the specific sensitizing antigen and subsequently examined for delayed hypersensitivity skin responses at the test site.

To measure pre-existing cell-mediated reactions, patients are usually skin tested with a variety of common ubiquitous microbial antigens (e.g., tuberculin (PPD), candida antigen, trichophyton, mumps, strep-tokinase-streptodornase (SK-SD), etc.). If a patient exhibits no delayed skin responses to any of five such antigens, that patient may be anergic in T cell responses. If the patient shows several positive skin test responses, it can only be assumed that the patient is not sensitized to those antigens which elicit no response. The latter antigens may then be used as sensitizing antigens (as DNCB or KLH) in determining whether that patient is able to form new cell-mediated immunities (CMI).

The capacity to reject a skin allograft is a sensitive test of an individual's capacity to mount a CMI response. Susceptibility to certain infectious diseases may be an indicator of deficient CMI, since individuals with deficient CMI tend to have a greater incidence of infections caused by fungi, viruses and facultative intracellular bacteria. Another indication of cell-mediated immune capability is the presence of an abundant cell population in the thymic-dependent areas of the lymph nodes.

ANTIGEN-SPECIFIC T CELL RECEPTORS

Controversy exists as to the nature of the antigen-specific T cell receptor. Some investigators have found in mice that L chains are part of the T cell receptor while others have found mu chains as a portion of the T cell receptors. It has even been argued that certain common amino acid sequences in the L chains and mu chains may account for this discrepancy. Most investigators do not find known immunoglobulin structures associated with the T cell receptor. Some investigators have suggested that the T cell receptors may be composed entirely of L chains or that the L chains are associated with a unique class of H chain in the T cell membrane. The number of immunoglobulin receptors on B cells is estimated to be about 10^5, while the number (*if existing*) on T cells would be below the limits of detection by direct technics (not exceeding 10^3). While the existence of T cell receptors is not doubted, their immunoglobulin nature is.

A chemical definition of the T cell receptor will greatly aid our understanding of T cell responses which mediate cell-mediated immunity and helper functions in antibody formation. T and B cell collaborative responses are essential in the formation of most of our classes of antibody immunoglobulins. A T-to-T cell interaction with antigen may even be necessary for the proliferation of detectable antigen-specific T cells.

TRANSFERABILITY OF CMI

Cell-mediated immune phenomena such as delayed skin reactivity *cannot* be transferred by sera from sensitive to nonsensitive individuals. CMI can be transferred with populations of lymphoid cells (*adoptive transfer*) containing antigen-reactive T cells (sensitized cells) or with certain extracts or products of these sensitized T cells. For example, an *antigen-liberated transfer factor* of large molecular weight is a lymphokine capable of conferring specific antigen-reactivity to other lymphocytes. Approximately 20 years ago, Lawrence described a low molecular weight factor (less than 10,000) present in the dialysate of cell lysates prepared by repeated freezing and thawing of peripheral blood leukocytes. *Lawrence type dialyzable transfer factor*, although resistant to the action of trypsin and ribonuclease, has been shown to be nucleotide and polypeptide in nature. Originally, Lawrence's dialyzable transfer factor was prepared from PPD skin test positive donors and was able to convert nonsensitive recipients to PPD skin sensitivity within 24 hours after injection. Such specific delayed hypersensitivity remained for 18 months to 2 years in the recipients. As yet, the mode of action of such dialyzable transfer factors (DTF) is not known. The amount of nucleotides contained in DTF is too small for the material to function as a messenger RNA. The prevailing opinion is that the low molecular weight transfer factor, in some manner, acts as a derepressor of gene function specifying specific antigen reactivity by certain subpopulations of T cells. Dialyzable transfer factors are not consistently found in dialysates of peripheral blood lymphocytes from host species other than man. A ribonuclease-sensitive RNA extract of human lymph node cells was found by Thor and Dray to transfer donor-type delayed sensitivities to the lymphoid cells of nonsensitive individuals in cell culture.

INDUCTION OF CELL-MEDIATED IMMUNITY

The induction of cell-mediated immune responses is favored when a complex lipid-containing antigen is used in conjunction with an adjuvant. Apparently, the chemical complexity of the antigen favors T cell interactions; the intrinsic lipids localize the antigen in the thymus-dependent area of the regional lymph nodes draining the injection site (see Chapter 7) and the adjuvant favors T cell participation (see Chapter 2). For example, contact sensitivities such as poison ivy are supposedly induced following binding of the caustic oil with host protein in the skin. The subcutaneous fat may exert an adjuvant action upon the immunogenicity of such a hapten-carrier complex. Consequently, a T cell response is initiated in the regional lymph nodes.

Demonstrable cell-mediated immune phenomena do not occur in response to thymic-dependent antigens unless an adjuvant is employed. Mackaness and associates have noted that small intravenous doses of a thymic-dependent antigen (sheep erythrocytes) stimulate detectable delayed hypersensitivity in mice. However, large doses of the same antigen given intravenously induced only antibody formation. From this and other evidence they concluded that a product of the antigen-antibody interaction blocks the activated T cells which mediate delayed hypersensitivity without interfering with helper cells. Evidence from other laboratories also indicates that T cell helper function is separable from T cell mediator function.

CELL-MEDIATED IMMUNE RESPONSES IN VIVO

In a simplistic fashion in vivo cell-mediated immune responses may be compared with the host inflammatory responses: a small to moderate response is beneficial to the host while an extensive response is detrimental to the host.

The unfavorable aspects of cell-mediated immune responses under natural circumstances probably occur rarely and more often as a consequence of infectious disease. A severe, but fortunately rare, response is a systemic delayed hypersensitivity reaction. Certain infectious disease agents such as viruses *may* alter self antigens to induce autoimmune disease states which are initiated by cell-mediated immune responses (see Chapter 10). Even though allograft rejection and graft-versus-host (GVH) phenomena are mediated by T cells and may lead to lethality in the host, they are not the result of natural circumstances. Some investigators feel that cell-mediated immune responses against certain microbial agents contribute to granuloma formation.

The walling-off of microbial invaders by granuloma formation may be considered beneficial to the host, e.g., the formation of a calcified tubercle. However, extensive granulomatous formations may exert an adverse effect on the host if these occur in vital organs, e.g., the gumma formations in the brain, heart, etc., seen in tertiary syphilis.

As Mackaness has shown, cell-mediated immune responses at the cellular level are beneficial to the host in ridding the infected host of facultative intracellular parasites and of certain viruses (see Chapter 8). This process probably involves circulating T cells interacting with microbial antigens in infected foci with the subsequent release of lymphokines and the activation of macrophages to heightened microbicidal activity (the "angry" macrophage).

SUGGESTED READINGS

Bloom, B. R., and Glade, P. R.: *In Vitro Methods in Cell-Mediated Immunity* (New York: Academic Press, 1971).

Coon, J., and Hunter, R.: Selective induction of delayed hypersensitivity by a lipid conjugated protein antigen which is localized in thymus dependent lymphoid tissue, J. Immunol. 110:183, 1973.

David, J. R.: Lymphocyte mediators of cellular hypersensitivity, N. Engl. J. Med. 288:143, 1973.

Good, R. A., Biggar, W. D., and Park, P. H.: Immunodeficiency diseases of man, in Amos, B. (ed.): *Progress in Immunology I* (New York: Academic Press 1971), p. 699.

Gottlieb, A. A., *et al.*: What is transfer factor, Lancet 2:822, 1973.

Humphrey, J. H., and White, R. G. (eds.): *Immunology for Students of Medicine* (3rd ed.; Philadelphia: F. A. Davis Co., 1970).

Jamieson, C. W., and Wallace, J. H.: Cytostasis of mouse and human monolayer cell cultures by normal, unstimulated lymphocytes, J. Immunol. 105:7, 1970.

Joklik, W. K., and Smith, D. T. (eds.): *Zinsser Microbiology* (15th ed.; New York: Appleton-Century-Crofts, 1972).

Katz, D. H., and Benacerraf, B.: The regulatory influence of activated T cells on B cell responses to antigen, Adv. Immunol. 15:1, 1972.

Lagrange, P. H., Mackaness, G. B., and Miller, T. E.: Influence of dose and route of antigen injection on the immunological induction of T cells, J. Exp. Med. 139:528, 1974.

Lawrence, H. S.: Mediators of cellular immunity, Transplant. Proc. 5:49, 1973.

Lawrence, H. S., and Landy, M. (eds.): *Mediators of Cellular Immunity* (New York: Academic Press, 1969).

Mackaness, G. B.: The J. Burns Amberson Lecture—The induction and expression of cell-mediated hypersensitivity in the lung, Am. Rev. Resp. Dis. 104:813, 1971.

Mackaness, G. B., *et al.*: Feedback inhibition of specifically sensitized lymphocytes, J. Exp. Med. 139:543, 1974.

Schlossman, S. F., *et al.*: Compartmentalization of antigen-reactive lymphocytes in desensitized guinea pigs, J. Exp. Med. 134:741, 1971.

Sorg, C., and Bloom, B. R.: Products of activated lymphocytes. I. The use of radiolabelling techniques in the characterization and partial purification of the migration inhibitory factor of the guinea pig, J. Exp. Med. 137:148, 1973.

Thor, D. E., and Dray, S.: The cell-migration-inhibition correlate of delayed hypersensitivity conversion of human nonsensitive lymph node cells to sensitive cells with an RNA extract, J. Immunol. 101:469, 1968.

Thor, D. E., and Dray, S.: Transfer of cell-mediated immunity by immune RNA assessed by migration-inhibition, in Freedman, H. (ed.): *RNA in the Immune Response*, Ann. N.Y. Acad. Sci. 207:355, 1973.

7 / Biology of the Immune Response

The existence of organized lymphoid tissues in a species correlates with its capacities to produce immunoglobulins and cell-mediated immune responses. Invertebrate species seem incapable of making "classic" immune responses, although bactericidal substances may be found in the hemolymph of certain crustaceans several days after injection of bacterial antigen and the earthworm has been shown capable of cell-mediated allograft rejection. When maintained in its natural environment, the California hagfish, a primitive cyclostome, is able to reject allografts and make antibodies to several antigens. This antibody response is the most primitive detected in a lower vertebrate which lacks both organized lymphoid tissues and thymus. The lamprey, a more advanced cyclostome which also makes a primitive immunoglobulin, lacks a true thymus but does possess an epithelial organ which may function as a thymus. Both cyclostomes make only a macroglobulin-like molecule. The more advanced cartilaginous and bony fishes possess a lymphoid thymus and make several classes of immunoglobulin molecules. The capacity to make immunoglobulins as well as cell-mediated immune responses is associated with all vertebrate species.

A pentameric macroglobulin similar to the IgM class of mammals has been found in representatives of the classes Aves, Reptilia, Amphibia and Chondrichthyes. An unusual tetrameric type of immunoglobulin has been found in the ray-finned fishes while the other subclass of bony fishes represented by the lungfish seems to have a pentameric type of IgM. A hexameric form of immunoglobulin is found in the clawed toad, an amphibian. The chicken has a low molecular weight immunoglobulin which is distinct from any immunoglobulin described in mammals. The duck possesses immunoglobulins with sedimentation coefficients of 7.8 and 5.7; the latter may be the 7.8S molecule lacking the Fc portion of H chains. Turtles, grouper and lungfish also contain low molecular weight immunoglobulins (5S to 6S). However, 7S immunoglobulins containing polypeptide chains similar to the human immunoglobulins are also found in chickens and amphibians.

Evidence for both the alternate complement pathway and terminal components of complement has been found in several invertebrate species, e.g., in the hemolymph of the horseshoe crab and the sepunculid worm. In the lamprey, no classic complement pathway was found and evidence for the alternate pathway was not sought. The sera of several higher fishes, e.g., lemon and nurse sharks, contain the components of the classic complement system. The two-limbed immune response as well as the complement system evolve phylogenetically as does the complexity of vertebrate forms.

ONTOGENY

The two limbs of the immune response in avian species serve as the model against which the human immune response is studied. In the chicken, the thymus is responsible for the maturation of cell-mediated immune (T cell) functions and the bursa of Fabricius, a cloacal lymphoid organ, is responsible for the maturation of the B lymphocyte-mediated immunoglobulin production. In the human, a well-developed thymus exists but no single organ comparable to the bursa of Fabricius has been found. Many investigators feel that the gut-associated lymphoid tissues (GALT) serve this function in the human (Figure 7–1). In chickens, at approximately 14 days of embryonation in the absence of antigens, B lymphocyte differentiation occurs in the bursa and IgM-containing cells are detected. Approximately 7 days later, IgG-containing cells can be found in the bursa. These cells then seed the peripheral lymphoid organs. If the bursa of Fabricius is ablated before 17 days of embryogenesis, the chickens are incapable of antibody synthesis upon hatching. The peripheral lymphoid tissues of such chickens exhibit no germinal center development and contain no plasma cells.

In the human fetus, B lymphocyte development is initiated at approximately the same time as T cell development (i.e., in the fetal liver about 9 weeks into gestation). Using immunofluorescent technics to detect membrane-bound immunoglobulins, Cooper and associates found only IgM-staining cells in the liver of one 9.5-week-old fetus; both IgM- and IgG-staining cells were seen in the liver of another 9.5-week-old fetus. IgA-staining cells were first seen in 11.5-week-old fetuses. By 14.5 weeks of gestation the peripheral blood lymphocytes

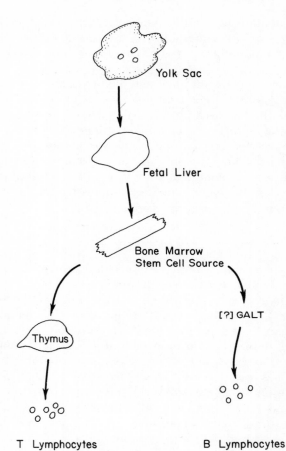

Fig. 7-1.—Ontogeny of the two limbs of the human immune response.

examined contained the same percentages of cells staining for IgM (8.8%), IgG (20%) and IgA (9.5%) as contained in the peripheral blood of term infants, children or adults (IgM = 4.4–13.9%; IgG = 8–30%; IgA = 3.7–12%). The spleens of these 14.5-week-old fetuses contained 19% IgM-staining cells, 20% IgG-staining cells and 9.5% IgA-staining cells. No cytoplasmic immunoglobulins were contained in the cells of the spleen, liver, thymus, bone marrow or blood of the 14.5-week-old fetuses. Such cytoplasmic immunoglobulins, indicative of active intracellular immunoglobulin synthesis, were seen later (15.5–23 weeks) and then only rarely.

Similar to the ontogenetic development of the B series of lymphocytes in the chicken, the human B cell system also appears to develop early in fetal life in a microenvironment supposedly free of antigenic stimuli. The first cells to appear bear IgM surface markers; cells bearing IgG membrane markers appear next, followed by cells bearing IgA surface markers. Since the appearance of these different cells is so constant in time from fetus to fetus, Lawton and colleagues argue that their development does not necessarily depend upon contact with antigens. Cells have been observed to switch from IgM to IgG synthesis; e.g., cultured myeloma cells contained surface-bound IgM and intracytoplasmic IgG. This phenomenon seen in cultured malignant cells may be a recapitulation of normal ontogenetic events.

In attempting to explain the fact that adult percentages of IgA-bearing cells are present in the 15-week-old fetus and yet adult levels of IgA are not usually seen until puberty, Lawton and associates suggest that active IgA synthesis requires some type of interaction of IgA-bearing cells with T cells. (Recall that the thymus involutes at the onset of puberty.) In mice, IgM responses are the least thymic-dependent of the three (IgM, IgG, IgA) immunoglobulin responses; IgG responses are more T cell-dependent than are IgM responses but less thymic-dependent than IgA responses.

Using autoradiographic technics, Miller and associates found IgE in human fetuses at 8.5 to 21 weeks of gestation. IgE-staining cells were present in fetal lung and liver at 11 weeks and in spleen at 21 weeks. In these studies IgE was not found in fetal heart, kidney, pancreas, adrenal, mesentery, thymus, bone marrow, blood, choroid plexus, yolk sac, placental umbilical cord or gastrointestinal tract.

Rowe and colleagues found IgD to be the predominant immunoglobulin on lymphocytes of the human newborn. Recently, Fu and associates noted that the majority of patients with chronic lymphatic leukemia have leukemic cells bearing IgD as well as IgM on their surface. In addition to these immunoglobulins, some cells carried free light chains. The significance of these observations is not yet clear.

The "primitive" B cell is referred to as a pre-bursal cell. Found in the blood islets of the yolk sac, in the fetal liver and in bone marrow, this cell is not yet immunologically competent. By some as yet undefined process, competence is conferred upon pre-bursal cells after traffic to the bursa in the chicken (or its equivalent lymphoepithelial site in mammals). The B_1 cell is a post-bursal cell found in the avian bursal medulla, in bone marrow and eventually in the spleen. The B_1 population contains cells of many antibody-forming potentials and is capable of long-term restoration of agammaglobulinemic, bursectomized animals. The B_2 post-bursal cell is present in the bursal medulla, in the germinal centers of lymph nodes and in periarteriolar accumulations in Malpighian corpuscles of spleen. B_2 cells are capable of synthesizing antibody but are not sufficiently differentiated for the secretion of large amounts of antibody. Following injection of antigen, the B_2 cells are present in the efferent lymph, the thoracic duct lymph and circulating blood. These cells probably bear antigen-specific receptors (membrane-bound immunoglobulins). The B memory cells, i.e., those antigen-specific B cells present in increased numbers following antigenic stimulation, are contained in the B_2 cell population. The post-bursal B_3 population of cells includes both cells identifiable as lymphocytes and plasma cells. Both types synthesize and secrete antibody globulins. B_3 cells are present in bone marrow, medullary cords of lymph nodes, red pulp of spleen, lamina propria of the gastrointestinal tract and secretory glands, and interstitial tissue of bone marrow. On occasion, B_3 cells may be seen in the peripheral blood and/or lymph.

At birth, the human infant is not a likely candidate for purposeful immunization. For one reason, the neonate contains maternal IgG as a result of placental transfer and those maternal antibodies may prevent the fetus from responding to specific antigens. Secondly, based on observations in animals, immunologic tolerance to some antigens may be readily induced in the neonate. And finally, certain experimental evidence indicates that neonatal macrophage function is immature. Purposeful immunization (vaccination) is not usually performed in the human infant until 2–3 months of age when most of the maternal IgG has been degraded.

In over 90% of healthy infants of normal birth weight, IgA can be detected in the tears within 10–20 days of life, while IgM has been found in infant tear specimens during the fourth week following birth. In infants of low birth weight the appearance of IgA in the tears is slightly delayed. If an infant has infective conjunctivitis, IgA is detectable in the tears as early as the third and fourth days of life. Normally, the synthesis of IgM, IgA and probably some IgG begins within the first 4–6 weeks of life.

IgM synthesis begins prenatally and adult serum levels are reached by 1–3 years of age. If, however, a fetus is infected in utero with certain viruses such as rubella, abnormal maturation of the immune mechanisms usually occurs. Such infected infants have elevated serum levels of IgM and IgA in the first days of life.

All children with congenital rubella infections have high levels of antibody to the rubella virus, but occasionally an IgG deficiency results which leads to an antibody deficiency syndrome.

Uhr and associates have shown that the human newborn can make antibody responses to some antigens but not others during the first month of life. Both premature and full-term infants were able to make antibody to a bacteriophage and cell-mediated immune responses to dinitrochlorobenzene (DNCB) during the first month of life. The premature or full-term newborn did not form detectable antitoxin to diphtheria and tetanus toxoids during the first month of life but was able to do so 4–10 weeks after birth. No attempts were made to assay maternal antibody specificities in these infants.

Usually, IgM and IgG serum concentrations reach adult levels at 2–3 years of age, while adult levels of IgA are present at about 12 years of age (puberty). Adult IgE levels apparently are reached sometime between 15–20 years of age.

Cell-mediated immune potential, as measured by the effect of the mitogen phytohemagglutinin on the thymic-dependent lymphocytes (T cells), is present in the human fetus and functional at birth. It is apparently this portion of the immune response which may be lost upon aging in certain inbred mice. Nakano and Braun restored the waning capacity of aging inbred mice to make antibody by injecting the mice with a synthetic polynucleotide. The mice were restored to the immunologic vigor of young adult mice of the same strain. Did the polynucleotide adjuvant function by prodding T cell activity so that T cell-dependent B cell responses occurred?

The concept of immune surveillance maintains that recognition of self from non-self antigens is a property of the T cell system. When self antigens are altered and the alteration is recognized immunologically, autoimmune processes may develop. When a malignant alteration occurs which is not recognized immunologically, malignancy may develop. Consequently, certain investigators have considered both autoimmunity and malignancy as a natural progression in the aging process of the human species. Virus-induced depression or derangement of T lymphocytes may afford an early expression of these diseases in certain members of the species. This topic is continued in Chapters 10 and 11.

THYMIC HUMORAL FACTOR

Cell-free thymic humoral factors from human and numerous animal species have been studied for their effects on the immune system. Thymic humoral factor has been found capable of restoring several immunologic responses in mice lacking thymuses. A lymphocytosis-producing factor of the thymic origin has been noted in humans and mice with chronic lymphoid leukemia. In thymectomized mice, thymosin (a protein or glycoprotein extract from calf thymus) restores certain CMI capacities (accelerated allograft rejection responses, prevention of wasting syndrome, increase in theta-positive cells and increased blastogenic responses by lymph node cells) yet does not appear to influence significantly the T cell capacity to function as "helper" in B cell responses.

T CELL RECEPTORS AND ROSETTE-FORMING CELLS

Mice immunized with sheep erythrocytes (SRBC's) form rosette-forming lymphoid cells. These cells bind SRBC's so that a rosette-like cell arrangement is seen microscopically, i.e., SRBC's clustered around lymphocytes. A portion of these rosette-forming cells in mice are undoubtedly B cells since they also form hemolytic plaques (mouse spleen cells secreting complement-binding IgM antibody for SRBC). However, most rosette-forming cells (RFC's) do not form plaques of 19S-globulin-producing cells; even by electronmicroscopy RFC's appear as nonsecretory cells. In immunized mice, RFC's are present in the spleen in greatly increased numbers 5 days after immunization. Although present in highest concentrations in the spleen, they are also present in all lymphoid organs of immunized mice. (RFC's are present in least numbers in the thymus.) The T cells forming rosettes bind fewer SRBC's than do B cells. Rosette formation may be inhibited by antisera to mouse immunoglobulins. The evidence that rosette-forming T cells are inhibited from binding SRBC only by anti-IgM (containing antibodies with specificities directed against the "hinge" region of the mu chain) or anti-light chain sera (especially by anti-kappa chain sera) has convinced some investigators that the T cell receptor is immunoglobulin in nature.

LYMPHOCYTE SURFACE MARKERS

Mouse Cell Markers

In the mouse, surface markers for B and T lymphocytes have been described. B cells possess a high density of surface immunoglobulin determinants and high densities of histocompatibility antigens, i.e., H-2 alloantigens. Receptors for the Fc portion of antibody are present on differentiated cells but not on mouse plasma cells while the MBLA marker (mouse bone marrow-derived lymphocyte antigen) appears to be present on the surfaces of both B lymphocytes and plasma cells. On the plasma cells of mice a unique alloantigen exists which is called PC (plasma cell) alloantigen.

Theta alloantigen is absent on mouse B cells but present on most peripheral T lymphocytes. In contrast to the B cell system, the T cells contain a low density of histocompatibility antigens and lack PC alloantigen, MBLA and receptors for the Fc region of antibody molecules. The possible presence of an Fc-like receptor on T cells has been described; mouse T cells bind cytophilic gamma globulin.

Human Cell Markers

B lymphocytes are characterized in both mouse and man by surface immunoglobulins and by receptors for aggregated immunoglobulins, antigen-antibody complexes and C3. Such receptors are detected by a rosette test in which erythrocytes are first coated with C3 or antibody and then reacted with suspensions of lymphoid cells. The coated erythrocytes attach to receptors on B cells; the B cell is seen with red cells clustered around it as a rosette.

A marker similar to the mouse theta antigen is being sought on human T cells. Wybran and Fudenberg use a rosette test for detecting human T cells in peripheral blood. Certain human lymphocytes will bind in vitro with washed, uncoated sheep erythrocytes. The mechanism of this nonimmune rosette reaction is not clear (although in other species the sheep red cell is a T cell-dependent antigen). Rosette-forming cells are decreased in number in patients with impaired cell-mediated immune capacities. Clinically, the nonimmune rosette test is being used as a T cell marker in the diagnosis and evaluation of various autoimmune and immunodeficiency diseases; in the estimation of the immunosuppressant effects of antilymphocyte sera (ALS); in measuring the efficacy of immunosuppressant drugs; and even to measure the thymosin-like activity in human serum.

A number of investigators have attempted to separate B and T lymphocytes in cell suspensions which have been passed through columns containing antigen bound to an insoluble matrix (for example, Sephadex G-200, Sepharose, or polyacrylamide beads [Bio-Gel]). By this method, only B cells from both unimmunized and immunized animals bind to the antigen. Wolfsky and colleagues observed that only one cell in 3×10^5 normal lymphocytes was bound to a column in which a hapten (azophenyl β-lactoside) was linked to Bio-Gel. When these specifically antigen-reactive cells together with T cells were transferred to irradiated recipient hosts, a 3000-fold increase in the B cells reactive only to this antigen occurred following stimulation with complete antigen (hapten-linked to carrier). These results support the clonal selection theory of antibody formation (see Chapter 3).

T cells appear unable to bind to simple antigens in such affinity columns. However, specifically reactive T cells may be removed from a suspension of lymphoid cells by exposure to complex cellular antigens. Edelman has developed a method for binding both T and B antigen-reactive cells. Antigen-coupled (derivatized) nylon fibers bind both antigen-reactive T and B cells from suspensions of mouse spleen cells.

NUTRITION AND THE IMMUNE RESPONSE

In nutritionally deprived animals, depression of host resistance to pyogenic and intracellular bacterial infection occurs, as does increased resistance to some viral infections and malignant tumors. Specific cell-mediated cytotoxic tumor responses remained intact in mice fed protein-deficient or protein-limited diets. In the same animals a profound depression in humoral antibody was noted. These observations suggest that such nutritionally deficient animals are more resistant to malignancy than are well-nourished animals.

FUNCTIONING IMMUNORESPONSIVENESS

A critical relationship exists between the three-dimensional conformation of an antigen and its capacity to trigger B cells. Thymus-independent antigens, such as pneumococcal polysaccharides and the lipopolysaccharide endotoxins of gram-negative enteric bacilli, stimulate mainly antibody responses of the IgM class. Apparently, most natural as well as many artificial antigens (hapten-carrier combinations) require the collaborative effect of T cells in the triggering of B cell responses (IgG). In responder strains of mice, early IgM antibody responses follow IgG responses to antigen, while nonresponder strains produce only IgM in response to the same antigen. Consequently, T cells seem to be necessary for B cells to be stimulated to IgG production, switching the response to a given antigen from IgM antibody synthesis to IgG antibody synthesis. Moreover, in the study of the antibody response to haptens, this T cell influence has been shown necessary for the emergence of B cells bearing high affinity receptors.

Kagnoff and colleagues question the thymus independence of any antigen. They suggest that the repeating polymeric nature of the so-called thymus independent antigens permits inductive interactions at very low levels of T cell cooperation. Since antibody responses to these antigens are mainly of the IgM class, Barthold and associates suggest that this occurs because B cells bearing specific IgM receptors are more likely to bind the polymeric antigen and be triggered than are

B cells carrying IgG or IgA type antigen receptors. In studying the response of mice to pneumococcal polysaccharide type III, they found small but significant numbers of IgG and IgA plaque-forming cells in addition to the IgM plaque-forming cells. Following inactivation of T cells (by treatment with antilymphocyte serum), the numbers of IgG and IgA plaque-forming cells increased at least 10-fold. Consequently, these investigators suggest that amplifier and suppressor T cells act in opposing manner to regulate the magnitude of the IgM response to the B cell system to pneumococcal polysaccharide type III. Baker and associates indicate that suppressor T cells limit the extent of B cell proliferation following immunization with type III polysaccharide.

In attempts to compare the effects of free antibody and cellular antigen receptors on the tertiary effects of antigen structure, Modabber and collaborators have studied an unusual antigen. The antigen examined is an inactive β-galactosidase-like substance produced by certain E. coli mutants. When this antigen is bound to free antibody it becomes enzymatically active. Modabber believes that the antibody-mediated activation involves only one alteration in the tertiary structure in the antigen which is called AMEF (antibody-mediated enzyme forming substance). When AMEF was bound to cell receptors it remained enzymatically inactive.

McDevitt and associates have found unexpectedly that low-responder mice do give rise to a population of IgG-bearing cells after primary antigenic stimulation but that the maturation into IgG secreting cells is not completed. The inability of low-responders to form circulating IgG type antibody to a given antigenic determinant results because the animals lack antigen-reactive T cells. These investigators feel that T cells are not involved in the switch from IgM to IgG receptors on B cells, but that T cells *are* involved in the process of stimulating B cells to proliferate and differentiate into IgG-producing cells.

Similar to inbred strains of mice and guinea pigs, the human species also appears to possess immune response (ImR) genes associated, in some manner, with the histocompatibility gene system. An association between HL-A haplotypes and IgE antibody responses has been noted. Marsh and associates have observed that the ability of ragweed-sensitive humans to respond to a minor antigenic determinant was associated with the presence of HL-A7. The determinant is labeled Ra_5 and has a molecular weight of 5200. Only 17% of individuals highly sensitive to ragweed reacted with Ra_5 determinant; these persons also possessed the HL-A7 gene.

Weigle has raised the question of whether immunocompetence

correlates in any manner with the capacity to induce unresponsiveness during fetal life. He cites the fact that tolerance to soluble antigens such as bovine serum albumin (BSA) in the rabbit is readily induced during the first 9 days after birth. Rabbits are capable of making antibody to BSA between the eighth and twenty-first day of life. Silverstein and co-workers were able to invoke antibody responses to some antigens in fetal lambs. The stimulating antigens were essentially soluble materials in adjuvants. For example, bacteriophage, horse ferritin and ovalbumin stimulated antibody responses in fetal lambs from 53 to 150 days of gestation. On the other hand, antibody responses to other antigens (diphtheria toxoid, *Salmonella typhosa* and bacillus Calmette-Guérin) did not develop during the fetal existence of the lamb.

Immune tolerance appears to be more easily induced when "foreign" soluble serum proteins are used as tolerizing antigen (tolerogen) than when particulate complex antigens such as bacteria or viruses are used as antigen. Particulate antigens are rapidly phagocytized from the circulation; because of their particulate nature, they do not equilibrate effectively between intravascular and extravascular compartments. Consequently, little opportunity exists for them to reach all antigen-reactive cells.

T lymphocytes are able to suppress immune responses both specifically and nonspecifically. Ha and Waksman have recently shown that thymic T cells, which had not yet emigrated out of the thymus, were antigen-reactive and able to acquire suppressor function. Suppressor ability was examined when these cells were reexposed to specific antigen in syngeneic recipient rats at peripheral sites. Based on these and other observations, they suggest that such an active thymocyte response is necessary in the establishment of tolerance to antigens including self antigens. Consequently, autoimmunization would occur when such cells are reduced in number. Consistent with this reasoning is the observation of Barthold and colleagues that suppressor T cell function declines with age in female NZB mice. These animals naturally develop autoimmune disease upon aging. The suppressor role of T cells may be as important as are their amplifier activities.

Watson suggests that high molecular weight glycoproteins are the effector molecules regulating the development and function of myeloid and lymphoid cells. For example, antigen-activated T cells release glycoproteins which are either stimulators (substances with a molecular weight of 150,000, and do not appear to be immunoglobulin) or suppressors (substances with a molecular weight of 10,000–20,000) of B cell responses in vitro. Experimentally, suppressor or stimulator production depends upon the concentration of T cells and the antigen used. It is unknown whether the cells which produce stimulator and suppressor activities are the same or different.

TWO-SIGNAL MODEL OF INDUCTION OF IMMUNE RESPONSES

The conceptual model of Bretscher and Cohn suggests that immunocompetent cells need to receive two membrane signals for activation to proliferative stages. Antigenic determinants bound to specific membrane-bound immunoglobulin receptors on a given B cell effect a conformational change in the B cell membrane; this is signal one at the B cell membrane. If no other signal is received that particular B cell becomes tolerant upon subsequent encounters with specific antigen. However, if a second signal is received on the B cell membrane to which antigen is bound, then the cell is induced to proliferate and subsequently produce antibody. Recent evidence indicates that the second signal may in fact be a soluble factor released by T cells reacting with antigen. T cells may interact with the same antigen or even with unrelated antigens to supply the trigger for B cell responses. T cells need not interact with the same antigenic determinant sites as do B cells. This contention is supported by observations that certain immunologic adjuvants exert their effect on B cell responses by activating T lymphocytes. In this two-signal model, it is presumed that T cells may collaborate with one another in inducing conformational changes in T cell membranes and subsequent cell proliferation to the level of detectable cell-mediated responsiveness.

The two-signal model allows a reinterpretation of the observations of Parish. The natural antigen flagellin requires T cell collaboration with B cells in the production of detectable serum antibody. However, polymerized flagellin does not. Polymerized flagellin alone activates B cells to antibody production. The large polymer of flagellin as it is presented to B cells may actually bind to *two* separate immunoglobulin receptors in the membrane and, thus, provide both signals one and two to the membrane. Acetoacetylated flagellin appears only to activate T cell responses to native flagellin. In this latter situation one might speculate that the heavily acetoacetylated flagellin is unrecognizable to B cells containing receptors for native flagellin but is recognized by certain T cells which then proliferate.

Coon and Hunter localized the I^{125}-labeled lipid-conjugated BSA (dodecanoic-BSA) in the thymic-dependent areas of guinea pig lymph nodes, while I^{125}-labeled BSA was localized only in the germinal centers (B cell areas). The enhanced capacity of hapten-conjugated proteins to stimulate cell-mediated immunity to the carrier protein and antibody to the hapten portion of the complex has led to several conclusions, namely, that the antigenic determinants stimulating B cell responses are either different from those stimulating T cell responses or are smaller. Actually both of these alternatives are possible. It has been suggested that the conjugated haptens block small B cell determinants of antigen but leave unaltered the conformation of the T cell determinants of the antigen complex. The plant mitogens, concanavalin A and phytohemagglutinin, in soluble form selectively activate T lymphocytes although they bind equally well to B lymphocytes. However, if these same mitogens are linked covalently to solid phase substances, they are capable of stimulating the proliferation of B cells.

The effect of macrophage-bound antigen must not be overlooked. Certain investigators have argued that cytophilic antibody held on macrophages may, after interaction with antigen, function as a T cell in collaborative B cell responses. Even when antigen is bound to dead macrophages, T cells are activated by such complexes and are then able to collaborate with B cells in inducing antibody formation to that antigen. In in vitro systems of antibody synthesis, certain investigators refer to macrophages as the glass-adherent cells or even as the A cells. Cohen and Paul have indicated that the macrophage-associated cytophilic antibody determines the antigen sensitivity of the system by permitting macrophages to bind larger amounts of antigen when antigen is present in low concentration. Consequently, this results in a more efficient stimulation of T cells.

The stimulating effect of *Bordetella pertussis* as an immunologic adjuvant appears to act on B cells directly when large doses of antigen are employed. When smaller doses of antigen are used, *B. pertussis* amplifies the antibody response via T cell mediation. Studying the adjuvant effect of *Corynebacterium parvum* on a T cell-independent antigen, Howard and associates suggested that both adjuvant and suppressive activities of this bacterium on B cell responses are probably mediated by activated macrophages. Also, *C. parvum* appears to be a potent stimulator of the reticuloendothelial system.

The inter-relationships between the B and T lymphocyte systems and the reticuloendothelial macrophage appear to exert mutual interactions which are, as yet, only partially understood. Dukor and Hartmann suggest that C3 bound to B cells may serve as the second signal for B cell activation. Since a T cell-dependent B cell response, i.e., antibody formation, was inhibited in animals in which C3 was depleted by cobra venom while T cell responses per se were not, they suggest that antigen-activated T cells may release C3-cleaving proteases into their microenvironment.

T cell-independent antigens are polymerized flagellin, lipopolysaccharide of *E. coli,* pneumococcal capsular polysaccharides, levan, polyvinylpyrolidone and haptens coupled to dextran (but not haptens coupled to protein). Each of these antigens alone can induce formation of IgM class of antibody. As cited previously, these are polymeric antigens with a rigid structural backbone and possess multiple valencies. Such structures can bind to multiple sites on B cells, i.e., can cross-link the immunoglobulin receptors. These same antigens are capable of activating and converting C3 in serum. Recall that some of these substances, e.g., dextran, pneumococcal polysaccharide and lipopolysaccharide, are capable of activating the alternate complement pathway via C3 (see Chapter 4). C3 receptors are present on B cells. C3 may also be activated by proteases released from either antigen-activated or antigen-stimulated T cells, or from macrophages, or by complexes of IgM and antigen.

MOBILITY OF LYMPHOCYTE SURFACE ANTIGENS AND RECEPTORS

Immunoglobulin receptors can be removed from the membrane of B cells by treatment with divalent anti-immunoglobulin antibody. B lymphocytes so treated demonstrate new surface immunoglobulin receptors after 4 hours. Antibody to the immunoglobulin receptors causes a redistribution of the receptors from a diffuse, patchy arrangement in the membrane to a polar, cap-like position. Pinocytotic vesicles have been shown underlying the "cap" in cells labeled in the cold. Immunoglobulin redistribution appears to be followed by pinocytosis of the membrane molecules. Multivalent (but not monosubstituted) hapten conjugates are also capable of inducing cap formation in suspensions of living lymphocytes. After binding with antigen, the surface immunoglobulin receptor can either be internalized pinocytotically by the lymphocyte or drop off the membrane. In the mouse, with sheep erythrocyte antigen, cap formation has been observed for rosette-forming B cells and theta-positive T cells. In the T lymphocyte rosettes the position of the theta antigen was shown to be distinct from the antigen receptor in that it did not move in the formation of the cap but remained distributed in the membrane. Capping of mouse membrane antigens (θ, TL and H-2) has been demonstrated in the presence of specific antibody to each antigen.

As yet, no correlation seems to exist between cap formation and immunogenic triggering by antigen.

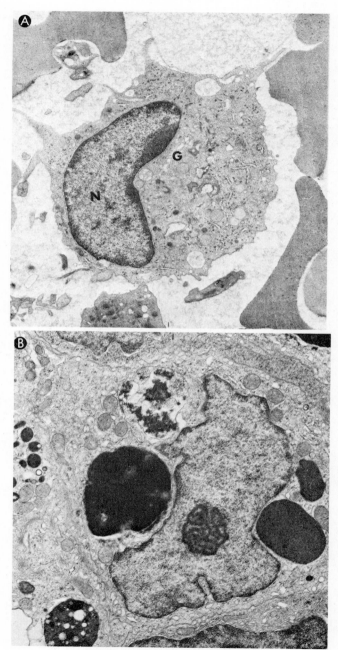

Fig. 7-2.—See legend on facing page.

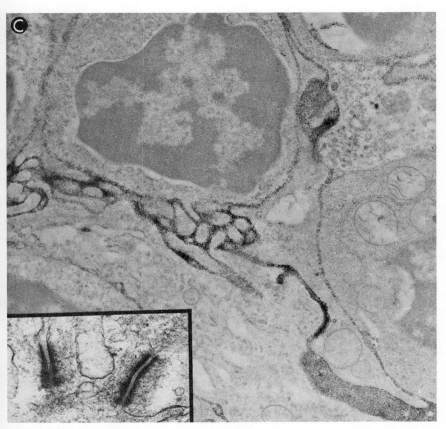

Fig. 7–2.—Monocyte and macrophage. **A**, the monocyte has a horseshoe-shaped nucleus (*N*). Its cytoplasm is more abundant than in the lymphocyte, shows a better developed Golgi complex (*G*) and numerous vesicles of various sizes as well as lysosomal granules. Two distinct types of macrophages possibly involved in the immune response are present in lymphoid organs. The first of these appears to be derived from the circulating blood monocyte and is known as the tingible body macrophage, **B**. Its name is derived from the fact that deeply staining phagocytized nuclear fragments and other particulate materials are found in its cytoplasm. The second type, present only in the germinal centers of the follicles, is known as the dendritic macrophage, **C**, because of its numerous long cytoplasmic extensions (dendrites), which interdigitate with similar extensions from neighboring macrophages, forming desmosome-like attachments (*insert*). These dendrites form a large surface area to which soluble antigens can adhere, as seen in this electronmicrograph of a portion of a germinal center of an experimental animal injected with the enzyme horseradish peroxidase. This tracer antigen can be seen along the membranes lining the dendritic processes.

By manipulating experimental conditions, certain substances (antilymphocyte serum and plant mitogens) can induce cap formation but not stimulation or stimulation and not cap formation. Simple ligand-receptor, i.e., antigen-antibody, interaction appears insufficient to trigger the lymphocyte. Triggering seems to require multivalent binding. For example, univalent anti-immunoglobulin or antilymphocyte sera (Fab fragments) are incapable of stimulating lymphocytes, while the F(ab')$_2$ fragments and whole antibody molecules can; the monomeric form of mitogenic phytohemagglutinin does not stimulate lymphocytes yet dimeric phytohemagglutinin does. Raff and DePetris argue that since polymeric antigens such as the bacterial endotoxins, polymerized flagellin or pneumococcal capsular polysaccharides can activate B cells directly to produce antibody, antigens which cannot bind multivalently to B cells may require participation of T cells and/or macrophages.

CELLULAR INTERACTIONS

As discussed in Chapter 2, the role of the macrophage in the induction of immune responses is difficult to define precisely. However, evidence indicates that macrophages and the B and T lymphocytes interact in various regulatory ways. Two types of macrophages which possibly function in the induction of the immune response are shown in Figure 7–2.

Potent stimulators of the reticuloendothelial system such as *C. parvum,* described previously, function as adjuvants in immune responses to other antigens. The adjuvant effect of *C. parvum* on B cell responses in mice to a thymic-independent antigen (pneumococcal polysaccharide) is indirect and probably mediated via activated macrophages. Although it has been shown that *C. parvum*-activated macrophages display an inhibitory effect on T cells which may have lower thresholds for activation by antigen than do B cells, factors released by these same activated macrophages have been postulated to stimulate B cells. In other words, factors released by activated macrophages may inhibit T cells while stimulating B cells. It is of interest to recall that macrophages can be activated by a lymphokine released by sensitized T cells in the presence of specific antigen. Thus, a T cell interacting with a thymic-dependent antigen may activate macrophages which, in turn, "shut off" further T cell activity while stimulating B cells to respond to antigen.

Both B and T lymphocytes have been shown to carry immunologic memory. Populations of memory cells were thought to contain both long-lived and short-lived lymphocytes, but more recently were shown to be relatively long-lived in the rat. Both types of memory cells cooperate in the induction of secondary antibody responses to a variety of antigens in rats and mice and are capable of recirculation from blood to lymph.

IMMUNOLOGIC DEFICIENCY DISEASES

We would probably not be at our present level of comprehension of the biology of the immune response if the immunodeficiency diseases had not been recognized. Primary immunodeficiency diseases are extremely rare in occurrence. These diseases are usually genetically determined anomalies but may be the result of developmental defects in the human fetus. Malignancies occur with greater frequency in all forms of primary immune deficiency diseases of man. Secondary immunodeficiency states arise following an interference with the lymphoreticular system by certain infectious agents or malignancy.

Primary Immunodeficiency Diseases

B CELL DEFECTS.—From an historical point of view, a defect in the B cell system was the first immunodeficiency state noted. Described in 1952 by Bruton and now bearing his name, Bruton's agammaglobulinemia is transmitted as a sex-linked (X-linked) trait. Affected children are not able to make much, if any, antibody following immunization. Consequently, they are unable to form plasma cells. Although their numbers of peripheral blood leukocytes are normal, they lack cells bearing surface immunoglobulins. (Normally 70–80% of human peripheral blood lymphocytes are T cells. B cells in the circulation may be identified by their surface immunoglobulins and/or C3 receptors.) They exhibit normal cell-mediated immune responses as shown by good protective host immunity to most viral pathogens, the ability to reject skin allografts, and the capacity to develop delayed type hypersensitive responses to poison ivy, chemicals and microbial antigens such as diphtheria toxoid and mumps virus. The thymuses of several of these children appeared similar in size and morphology to those of normal children at the same age. Because of maternal antibodies in their circulation, these infants are only occasionally ill before 6 months of age; after this time, however, they display marked susceptibilities to pyogenic bacterial pathogens (pneumococci, meningococci, streptococci and Pseudomonas) as well as to "viral" hepatitis. Patients are successfully maintained by treatment with antibiotics and routine administration of human gamma globulin. Children with Bruton's agammaglobulinemia are more prone to develop leukemias than are normal children.

Other types of agammaglobulinemias may also be transmitted as X-linked, autosomal recessive, or even autosomal dominant traits.

Probably the more frequent B cell deficiencies encountered in the human population are the selective immunoglobulin deficiencies. Of these, the most common is a selective deficiency of the IgA system. Children with selective IgA deficiency may exhibit either no clinical manifestations or frequently experience sinopulmonary and gastrointestinal infections.

T CELL DEFECTS.—There are several immune deficiences in which the thymic-dependent immune responses do not develop. In infants with DiGeorge's syndrome, the epithelial anlagen derived from the third and fourth pharyngeal pouches do not develop. This syndrome seems to be a developmental rather than a hereditary defect in which development of the parathyroid glands, calcitonin-producing thyroid cells, and epithelial thymus fails to occur. Since these infants display neonatal tetany it is possible to recognize and effectively treat this defect. In the few immunologic observations made in affected children at a few months of age, they have displayed normal or supranormal immunoglobulin levels, normal antibody responses to some antigens and normal plasma cell development. Lymph nodes show normally developed primary follicles and germinal centers, but thymic-dependent paracortical areas of the lymph nodes are depleted or lymphocytes (T cells). The peripheral blood lymphocytes of these children contain no T lymphocytes. Clinically, infants with T cell system deficiencies are prone to frequent infections by fungi, facultative intracellular parasites, and many viruses (measles, vaccinia virus, etc.). These children can be restored to normal immunologic vigor with a functioning T cell system following transplantation of human fetal thymus tissue. It is desirable that the donor tissue be histocompatible.

COMBINED B AND T CELL DEFECTS.—Infants with *Nezelof's syndrome* (heritable thymic aplasia) display normal parathyroid function but lack thymus-dependent immunologic functions. *Lymphopenic agammaglobulinemia* syndrome (Swiss type agammaglobulinemia) is transmitted as either an autosomal recessive or an X-linked characteristic. In this syndrome, the bone marrow source of lymphoid cell precursors fails to develop normally. Consequently, both T cell and B cell systems are absent. The thymuses of such infants are found high in the neck region and show arrested development, i.e., are composed of only epithelial cells. The peripheral blood, bone marrow and lymphoid organs display a marked absence of lymphocytes and plasma cells. Usually, infants with this genetic disease rarely survive beyond

12 months of age and succumb to either infection or malignancy. Such infants are unable to mount either antibody or cell-mediated immune responses. The first attempts to reconstitute the immune systems of such children were disastrous: the donor lymphocytes initiated fatal graft-versus-host reactions (see Chapter 11). In 1968 and 1969, restorations of a normally functioning immune system were achieved in several infants in which the HL-A antigens of donor lymphoid cells and recipient tissues were matched.

Combined immunodeficiency disease may also result from a *deficiency in adenosine deaminase (ADA)*. This enzymatic defect apparently prevents the lymphoid system from developing. Green and Chan suggest that the absence of adenosine deaminase may be the result of pyrimidine starvation induced by adenosine nucleotides in lymphoid cells; the increased concentrations of adenosine nucleotides might either kill or prevent the lymphoid cells from proliferating.

Lymphopenic dysgammaglobulinemia is also a dual-system immunodeficiency state inherited as either a sex-linked or sex-limited characteristic. Infants with this genetic deficiency cannot survive unless transplanted with histocompatible lymphoid cells and exhibit the same immunodeficiencies as do children with lymphopenic agammaglobulinemia. The lymphopenic dysgammaglobulinemia patient exhibits slight lymphoid system development in that the thymus, although small and poorly developed, has descended into the mediastinum, and the bone marrow contains a "normal" number of cells which appear morphologically as small lymphocytes. However, all peripheral lymphoid tissues exhibit marked deficiencies of small lymphocytes. Certain of these children have been observed to produce small quantities of one or another immunoglobulin. It is of interest to note that in the few male infants with these deficiency syndromes transplanted with histocompatible lymphoid cells from a sibling (usually a sister), all immunoresponsive cells are of the donor (female) karyotype.

In the multisystem sex-linked recessive *Wiskott-Aldrich syndrome,* the primary immunodeficiency state resides in the child's inability to process polysaccharide antigens as well as a marked deficiency in the production of platelets. Consequently, these children lack or possess only low concentration of IgM. (Recall that polysaccharide antigens are T cell-independent and directly stimulate antigen-reactive B cells to produce IgM.) Thus, isoagglutinins (anti-A and/or anti-B) are absent in their sera although serum concentrations of IgA and IgG are normal. Secondary to the inability to handle polysaccharides immunologically, these children display a progressive deficiency of cell-mediated immunities; they are susceptible to a wide array of microbial agents (bacteria, viruses and fungi) and are extremely prone to develop a wide variety of lymphoid malignancies (lymphoma, leukemia, carcinomas of the gastrointestinal tract and epitheliomas). In 1968, Bach and associates achieved a long-lasting bone marrow transplant in a male child from a female sibling matched for HL-A antigens but mismatched for ABO antigens. Therapeutically, the immunologic defects of this child have been corrected.

Ataxia telangiectasia is another multisystem genetic deficiency disease involving not only both limbs of the immunologic system but also the musculoskeletal system. Clinically, these children undergo repeated sinopulmonary infections. About 60% of patients lack both secretory and serum IgA, and they, also, undergo a progressive loss of cell-mediated immune capacity. The role of IgA and IgE deficiencies in this particular syndrome is intriguing yet unclear. Certain of these patients with sinopulmonary disease possess normal amounts of IgA but lack IgE. Good and associates observed that patients with genetically determined complete absence of IgA do not have recurring or progressive sinopulmonary infections when they possess normal amounts of IgE. Observations such as these suggest an undefined but intimate relationship between the normal functions of IgA and IgE systems and possibly in the capacity to form IgA, IgE and T cell responses. The range of malignancies encountered in these children is similar to that seen in Wiskott-Aldrich patients.

The World Health Organization now routinely publishes additions to the list of human immunodeficiency diseases. Our knowledge of the functioning immune system continues to grow, partly because of the astute observations of clinicians in the recognition of the various aberrations in human immunocompetency. Many more primary immunodeficiency diseases exist than are described here.

Primary genetic deficiency diseases which influence immunologic reactivity involve genetic deficiencies of the complement system (see Chapters 4 and 10) and of the host phagocytic cells.

PHAGOCYTIC CELL DEFICIENCIES.—Chronic granulomatous diseases of childhood are sex-linked or autosomal recessive traits and involve monocytes and polymorphonuclear neutrophils. These cells exhibit a deficiency in energy metabolism (hexose-monophosphate shunt) and also a deficiency in microbicidal activity. Consequently, affected children are chronically infected.

Chediak-Higashi syndrome is an abnormality of granule morphology and lysosomal function. Thus, children with this genetic disease also exhibit deficiencies in phagocytic cell capabilities and are chronically infected. The incidence of malignancy in children with primary immunologic and phagocytic diseases is higher than in normal children. The spectrum of infectious diseases seen in these various deficiency states has aided our comprehension of the mechanisms of protective host immunity.

Individuals with dual B and T cell system deficiencies do not survive unless immunologic restoration is accomplished. Death is attributed to either malignancy or infection early in life. Children with a B cell system deficiency encounter a high incidence of infections caused by pyogenic extracellular bacterial pathogens, hepatitis virus and *Pneumocystis carinii.* Individuals with T cell system deficiency display a high incidence of infections due to facultative intracellular parasites and viruses. Individuals with a leukocyte microbicidal deficiency are chronically infected by catalase-producing microorganisms such as Staphylococcus, Klebsiella, *Enterobacter aerogenes, Serratia marcescens, Candida albicans,* Aspergillus and Nocardia. Probably the most potent microbicidal substance produced by host phagocytes is a peroxide substance generated by the myeloperoxidase enzyme system (the genes for this system may be associated with those for the hexose-monophosphate shunt pathway). The deficient phagocytes are able to engulf microorganisms but lack the auxiliary energy provided by the hexose-monophosphate shunt mechanism to aid in either the digestion and/or generation of the myeloperoxidase killing system. Consequently, microorganisms which produce catalase are able to degrade any residual host cell peroxides and, in the absence of the complex myeloperoxidase-generating system, are able to persist within the host. (Chronic granulomatous disease of childhood is transmitted either as an X-linked trait or by other modes of inheritance.)

Myeloperoxidase (a lysosomal enzyme in polymorphonuclear neutrophiles [PMN's]) is actually lactoperoxidase. This enzyme functions in combination with H_2O_2 and a halide to form a markedly effective antimicrobial system. PMN's from individuals severely deficient in glucose-6-phosphate dehydrogenase and those from patients with chronic granulomatous disease fail to undergo the hexose-monophosphate shunt pathway and do not generate bactericidal hydrogen peroxide during phagocytosis.

Secondary Immune Deficiency States

Immunocompetence of the host organism undoubtedly involves mutual regulatory events (stimulation and inhibition) among macrophages and the T and B lymphoid cell systems. As yet, these events are ill-defined. Glimpses of these regulatory controls are seen when one or another of these cell types is malignantly transformed.

Human myeloma patients contain a serum factor which selectively depresses other B cell responses. Myeloma patients tend to have more infections induced by pyogenic bacteria and certain fungi than do normal individuals.

Patients with Hodgkin's disease may exhibit T cell-mediated immune anergy (inactivity) and the secondary infectious pattern in these patients confirms the T cell deficit. Only markedly anergic Hodgkin's disease patients will be frequently infected by facultative intracellular parasites such as *Mycobacterium tuberculosis, Salmonella typhimurium, Listeria monocytogenes,* Brucella, *Histoplasma capsulatum, Cryptococcus neoformans, Toxoplasma gondii* and viruses such as herpes zoster.

An infectious etiology is suspected in progressive multifocal leukoencephalopathy, a demyelinating syndrome associated with reticuloendothelial system diseases; this syndrome occurs commonly in association with Hodgkin's disease. However, both x-irradiation and drugs used in cancer chemotherapy are immunosuppressive in themselves.

In Hodgkin's disease, cell-mediated immune functions sometimes are absent during the later stages of the malignancy. The reason for this selective immunodeficiency is not clear. However, in patients successfully treated with x-irradiation and/or chemotherapy the return of T cell functions occurs. A possible explanation for the depression of T cells in this disease has been offered by Grifoni and colleagues who observed the existence of antilymphocyte antibodies in the sera of Hodgkin's disease patients. Experimentally, antilymphocyte serum (ALS) markedly depresses T cell functions, because circulating T cells are accessible. In the untreated early stage I Hodgkin's patient, no deficits in cell-mediated immunity (CMI) are evident. Sixty to seventy per cent of untreated patients in stages II, III and IV of active disease exhibit impaired CMI responses. Profound immunosuppression of both CMI and humoral immunity is seen only in patients with far-advanced terminal disease.

The pathologic hallmark of Hodgkin's disease is the Reed-Sternberg cell, a "malignant" histiocyte (tissue macrophage). Do such cells elaborate an immunosuppressive factor selective for T cell function or do they merely crowd out the T cells from their paracortical positions in lymphoid tissue? The derangement of T cell function in Hodgkin's disease closely parallels that of neonatally thymectomized animals.

In contrast to the Hodgkin's disease patient, humans with chronic lymphocytic leukemia appear to show first deficiencies in B cell responses. In line with this observation is the fact that patients with advanced malignancy have a high incidence of bacterial pneumonias. In these patients, the frequency of all bacterial infections is associated with hypogammaglobulinemia. In the terminal phases of disease, T cell responses also may be diminished. Aisenberg and Block observed marked increases of IgM-staining cells among peripheral blood lymphocytes from 25 patients with chronic lymphocytic leukemia (CLL) and three patients with chronic lymphosarcoma-cell leukemia, and on lymph node cells from three or four patients with lymphocytic lymphoma. They argue that these results favor the B cell origin of these particular leukemic cells and feel that the CLL lymphocyte is less likely a derepressed T cell. Recall that mu chain disease occurs in patients with long-standing CLL (see Chapter 3).

Harris and Sinkovics note that secondary neoplasms occur more frequently in patients with chronic lymphocytic leukemia than can be expected by chance alone. Coombs postulates that autoimmune hemolytic anemia, allergic vasculitis, thrombocytopenia purpura and lupus erythematosus may also occur in CLL patients.

Selective immunodeficiency associated with malignancy is often complex and need not lead to severe infectious disease. A woman with immunodeficiencies secondary to a follicular lymphoma of 14 years duration has been studied by Spitler, Levin and Fudenberg. The patient's life was not complicated by infectious disease even though she showed lymphopenia, no delayed hypersensitivity skin test responses to common microbial antigens, an inability to form new delayed type skin responses, and low serum globulin levels. Her resistance to infection was attributed to the presence of secretory IgA present in all mucous membrane secretions tested and to the fact that, although low in globulin content, her serum showed normal opsonizing abilities for *E. coli* and *S. aureus.*

In both lepromatous leprosy and sarcoidosis, deficits in cell-mediated immune capacity are seen. Although the etiology of sarcoidosis is unkown, that of leprosy (*M. leprae*) is well known. Upon pathologic examination of lymph node biopsies of the lepromatous patient, the thymus-dependent areas are depleted of lymphocytes but contain histiocytes teeming with the acid-fast *M. leprae.* As the T cells are depleted in both the lymph nodes and peripheral blood, the B cell system compensates in the lepromatous patient. Instead of comprising 10–20% of the peripheral blood lymphocytes, B cells are present in greatly increased numbers (60–85% of the total). Coincident with the increase in peripheral B cells is a marked decrease in T cells as measured by the lymphocytes which form spontaneous rosettes (same as nonimmune rosettes) with sheep erythrocytes. Patients with active lepromatous leprosy tend to have high serum IgM levels. One patient was even found with a large number of IgM-staining B cells in blood. Thus, it seems that when the T cell system is depressed, the thymic-independent B cells' response (IgM) is elevated. Again, we may ask: are the T cells selectively destroyed or suppressed by the infected histocytic cells or merely crowded out physically and unable to multiply? In the tuberculoid form of leprosy, the patients mount an effective CMI response. The paracortical areas of lymph nodes show hyperplasia and an absence of acid-fast mycobacteria. Turk and Bryceson have observed that once a patient is in the complete stage of commitment to lepromatous leprosy no drug treatment is able to reverse the disease to the tuberculoid form as can be done with patients in the borderline phase prior to lepromatous leprosy who are vigorously treated with drugs. The relationship between decreased CMI and high antibody levels is also seen in the condition known as erythema nodosum leprosum. In this state, red nodules occur in the skin which contain immunoglobulin and complement; this is seemingly an immune complex disease occurring in the lepromatous form of leprosy. Recently, Bullock and associates were able to impart lepromin sensitivity to anergic patients with lepromatous leprosy following injection of either small molecular weight transfer factor prepared from lepromin skin test positive donors or peripheral blood lymphocytes from these donors. This latter observation argues in favor of the possibility that the T cell system is not destroyed. Moreover, Park and colleagues injected allogenic human lymphoid cells into lepromatous leprosy patients and observed marked clinical improvement. Presumably macrophages were activated to kill the leprae bacilli.

Sarcoidosis, a generalized disease widely involving the lymphoid system, involves a relative depression of cell-mediated immunity with virtually intact antibody responses. Characteristic epithelioid granulomas may involve organs rich in reticuloendothelial cells, e.g., lymph nodes and spleen. Again, with depression of CMI in sarcoid patients elevated levels of serum globulins (IgA, IgM and IgG) are seen.

Unless the granulomatous lesion occurs in certain vital areas, sarcoidosis is a relatively mild disease. As in lepromatous leprosy, patients demonstrate anergy to other antigens. Sarcoid patients react to the Kveim antigen (tissue extract of sarcoid lesion). After a period of time, most sarcoid patients return to a normal immune responsive state and lesions usually undergo resolution. What is the disease? Why may it be self-limiting? Neither leprosy patients nor sarcoid patients are reported to be more susceptible to viruses or facultative intracellular parasites.

In attempts to uncover an explanation for the temporary suppression of delayed hypersensitivity in guinea pigs following administration of fairly large doses of antigen, Dwyer and Kantor support the concept of the existence of a humoral suppressant of cell-mediated immunity. Others have advocated the existence of humoral suppressants in states of generalized anergy seen in human granulomatous diseases such as leprosy, sarcoidosis, mucocutaneous candidiasis and syphilis. Immunologic deficiency in diffuse cutaneous leishmaniasis is a specific deficiency of CMI to Leishmania. The same may be true for individuals with any of these infectious diseases in which anergy to delayed type hypersensitivity responses to other antigens is seen. For example, Schulkind and associates have described a female child with CMI anergy to *C. albicans* whose circulating lymphocytes exhibited normal activation responses to allogeneic lymphocytes and to phytohemagglutinin.

Certain viruses are immunosuppressive of cell-mediated immune responses in man and animals. Following vaccination with attenuated yellow fever, polio or measles (rubeola) viruses, previously positive tuberculin skin reactions are depressed. Both rubeola and rubella viruses can readily be cultured from lymphoid cells during viral infection. Lactic dehydrogenase virus depresses CMI responses in mice. Wheelock and colleagues suggest that the selective immunosuppression of CMI by these agents may be related to the viral-induced lymphocytopenia. The phytohemagglutinin-induced blastogenic response of peripheral blood lymphocytes was inhibited or depressed in patients with rubeola, rubella or hepatitis virus infections, Burkitt's lymphoma, chronic lymphatic leukemia and infectious mononucleosis. Upon in vitro infection, the following viruses inhibited the phytohemagglutinin response of human lymphocytes: rubeola, rubella, herpes virus, Newcastle disease virus, vaccinia, vesicular stomatitis virus, poliovirus, ECHO virus, reo virus, Wart virus and serum from a hepatitis patient.

SUGGESTED READINGS

Acton, R. T., *et al.*: The carbohydrate composition of immunoglobulins from diverse species of vertebrates, J. Immunol. 109:371, 1972.

Aisenberg, A. C.: Malignant lymphoma, N. Engl. J. Med. 288:883, 1973.

Aisenberg, A. C., and Bloch, K. J.: Immunoglobulins on the surface of neoplastic lymphocytes, N. Engl. J. Med. 287:272, 1972.

134   Immunologic Fundamentals

Allansmith, M. R., McClellan, B. H., and Butterworth, M.: Individual patterns of immunoglobulin development in ten infants, J. Pediatrics 75:1231, 1969.

Armerding, D., and Katz, D. P.: Activation of T and B lymphocytes in vitro. I. Regulatory influence of bacterial lipopolysaccharide (LPS) on specific T-cell helper function, J. Exp. Med. 139:24, 1974.

Bach, J.-F.: Thymus dependency of rosette-forming cells, Contemp. Top. Immunobiol. 2:189, 1973.

Baehner, R. L., Johnston, R. B., Jr., and Nathan, D. G.: Comparative study of the metabolic and bactericidal characteristics of severely glucose-6-phosphate dehydrogenase-deficient polymorphonuclear leucocytes and leucocytes from children with chronic granulomatous disease, J. Reticuloendothel. Soc. 12.150, 1972.

Barthold, D. R., et al.: Regulation of the antibody response to type III pneumococcal polysaccharide. III. Role of regulatory T cells in the development of an IgG and IgA antibody response, J. Immunol. 112:1042, 1972.

Barthold, D. R., Kxsela, S., and Steinberg, A. D.: Decline in suppressor T cell function with age in female NZB mice, J. Immunol. 112:9, 1974.

Basten, A., and Howard, J. G.: Thymus independence, Contemp. Top. Immunobiol. 2:265, 1973.

Belcher, R. W., Connery, J. F., and Wanker, G. A.: In vitro inhibition of lymphocyte transformation by serum from patients with sarcoidosis, Clin. Res. 20:415, 1972.

Belohradsky, B. H., et al.: Meeting report of the second international workshop on primary immunodeficiency diseases in man, Clin. Immunol. Immunopathol. 2:281, 1974.

Bentwich, Z., et al.: Sheep red cell binding to human lymphocytes treated with neuraminidase; enhancement of T cell binding and identification of a subpopulation of B cells, J. Exp. Med. 137:1532, 1973.

Bergsma, D., and Good, R. A. (eds.): Immunologic Deficiency Diseases in Man, Birth Defects Original Article Series, Vol. IV, No. 1 (New York: The National Foundation – March of Dimes, 1968).

Bianco, C., Patrick, R., and Nussenzweig, V.: A population of lymphocytes bearing a membrane receptor for antigen-antibody-complement complexes. I. Separation and characterization, J. Exp. Med. 132:702, 1970.

Blanden, R. V.: Modification of macrophage function, J. Reticuloendothel. Soc. 5:179, 1968.

Blankenship, W. J., et al.: Serum gamma-M globulin responses in acute neonatal infections and their diagnostic significance, J. Pediatr. 75:1271, 1969.

Bretscher, P.: Hypothesis: A model for generalized autoimmunity, Cell. Immunol. 6:1, 1973.

Bretscher, P. A., and Cohn, M.: A theory of self-nonself discrimination, paralysis and induction involve the recognition of one and two determinants on an antigen, respectively, Science 169:1042, 1970.

Bullock, W. E.: Impairment of phytohemagglutinin (PHA) and antigenic induced DNA synthesis in leucocytes cultured from patients with leprosy, Clin. Res. 16:328, 1968.

Cohen, B. E., and Paul, W. E.: Macrophage control of time-dependent changes in antigen sensitivity of immune T lymphocyte populations, J. Immunol. 112:359, 1974.

Cohnen, G., et al.: Correspondence, B lymphocytes in Hodgkin's disease, N. Engl. J. Med. 288:161, 1973.

Coon, J., and Hunter, R.: Selective induction of delayed hypersensitivity by a lipid conjugated protein antigen which is localized in thymus dependent lymphoid tissue, J. Immunol. 110:183, 1973.

Cooper, M. D., et al.: Classification of primary immunodeficiencies, N. Engl. J. Med. 288:966, 1973.

Cooper, M. D., Lawton, A. R., and Kincade, P. W.: A developmental approach to the biological basis for antibody diversity, in Hanna, M. G., Jr. (ed.): Contemp. Top. Immunobiol. 1:33, 1972.

Drutz, D. J., Chen, T. S. N., and Lu, W.-H.: The continuous bacteremia of lepromatous leprosy, N. Engl. J. Med. 287:159, 1972.

Dukor, P., and Hartmann, K. U.: Hypothesis: Bound C3 as the second signal for B-cell activation, Cell. Immunol. 7:349, 1973.

Dwyer, J. M., Bullock, W. E., and Fields, J. P.: Disturbance of the blood T:B lymphocyte ratio in lepromatous leprosy, clinical and immunologic correlations, N. Engl. J. Med. 288:1036, 1973.

Dwyer, J. M., and Kantor, F. S.: Regulation of delayed hypersensitivity, failure to transfer delayed hypersensitivity to desensitized guinea pigs, J. Exp. Med. 137:32, 1973.

Edelman, G. M.: Antibody structure and molecular immunology, Science 180:830, 1973.

Farid, N. R., et al.: Rosette inhibition test for the demonstration of thymus-dependent lymphocyte sensitization in Graves's disease and Hashimoto's thyroiditis, N. Engl. J. Med. 289:1111, 1973.

Fu, S. M., Winchester, R. J., and Kunkel, H. G.: Occurrence of surface IgM, IgD, and free light chains on human lymphocytes, J. Exp. Med. 139:451, 1974.

Gajl-Peczalska, K. J., et al.: B lymphocytes in lepromatous leprosy, N. Engl. J. Med. 288:1033, 1973.

Gershon, R. F., et al.: Suppressor T cells, J. Immunol. 108:586, 1972.

Good, R. A., Biggar, W. D., and Park, B. H.: Immunodeficiency diseases of man, in Amos, B. (ed.): Progress in Immunology I (New York: Academic Press, 1971), p. 699.

Good, R. A.: Structure-function relations in the lymphoid system, Clin. Immunobiol. 1:1, 1972.

Gowans, J. L., and Uhr, J. W.: The carriage of immunological memory by small lymphocytes in the rat, J. Exp. Med. 124:1017, 1966.

Green, H., and Chan, T-S.: Pyrimidine starvation induced by adenosine in fibroblasts and lymphoid cells: Role of adenosine deaminase, Science 182:836, 1973.

Grifoni, V., et al.: Antilymph node antibodies in Hodgkin's disease (brief report), Boll. Ist. Sieroter. Milan. 48:75, 1969.

Ha, T.-Y., and Waksman, B. H.: Role of the thymus in tolerance. X. "Suppressor" activity of antigen-stimulated rat thymocytes transferred to normal recipients, J. Immunol. 110:1290, 1973.

Ha, T.-Y., Waksman, B. H., and Treffers, H. P.: The thymic suppressor cell. I. Separation of subpopulations with suppressor activity, J. Exp. Med. 139:13, 1974.

Hämmerling, G. J., Masuda, T., and McDevitt, H. O.: Genetic control of the immune response frequency and characteristics of antigen-binding cells in high and low responder mice, J. Exp. Med. 137:1180, 1973.

Hardy, J. B., et al.: Serum immunoglobulin levels in newborn infants. III. Some preliminary observations from a survey of cord blood levels in 2,600 infants, J. Pediatr. 75:1211, 1969.

Harris, J. E., and Sinkovics, J. G.: The Immunology of Malignant Disease (St. Louis, Mo.: C. V. Mosby Co., 1970).

Hecht, F., McCaw, B., and Koler, R. D.: Ataxia-telangiectasia-clonal growth of translocation lymphocytes, N. Engl. J. Med. 289:286, 1973.

Holmes, B., and Good, R. A.: Laboratory models of chronic granulomatous disease, J. Reticuloendothel. Soc. 12:216, 1972.

Howard, J. G., Christie, G. H., and Scott, M. T.: Biological effects of Corynebacterium parvum. IV. Adjuvant and inhibitory activities on B lymphocytes, Cell. Immunol. 7:290, 1973.

Hudson, L.: Review: Lymphocyte fractionation and purification, Curr. Titles Immunol. Transplant, Allergy 1:1, 1973.

Jerne, N. K.: The immune system, Sci. Am. 229:52, 1973.

Jondal, M., Holm, G., and Wigzell, H.: Surface markers on human T and B lymphocytes. I. A large population of lymphocytes forming nonimmune rosettes with sheep red blood cells, J. Exp. Med. 136:207, 1972.

Jose, D. G., and Good, R. A.: Quantitative effects of nutritional essential amino acid deficiency upon immune responses to tumors in mice, J. Exp. Med. 137:1, 1973.

Kagnoff, M. F., Billings, P., and Cohn, M.: Functional characteristics of Peyer's patch lymphoid cells. II. Lipopolysaccharide is thymus dependent, J. Exp. Med. 139:407, 1974.

Karnovsky, M. J., and Unanue, E. P.: Mapping and migration of lymphocyte surface macromolecules, Fed. Proc. 32:55, 1973.

Klebanoff, S. J., and Hamon, C. B.: Role of myeloperoxidase-mediated antimicrobial systems in intact leucocytes, J. Reticuloendothel. Soc. 12:170, 1972.

Lawton, A. R., Self, K. S., Royal, S. A., and Cooper, M. D.: Ontogeny of B-lymphocytes in the human fetus, Immunol. Immunopathol. 1:84, 1972.

Lay, W. H., *et al.*: Binding of sheep red blood cells to a large population of human lymphocytes, Nature 230:531, 1971.

Lee, S.-T., and Paraskevas, F.: Cell surface-associated gamma globulins in lymphocytes. IV. Lack of detection of surface γ-globulin on B-cells and acquisition of surface γ globulin by T-cells during primary response, J. Immunol. 109:1262, 1972.

Lerner, R. A., and Dixon, F. J.: The human lymphocyte as an experimental animal, Sci. Am. 228:82, 1973.

Levin, A. S., *et al.*: Wiskott-Aldrich syndrome, a genetically determined cellular immunologic deficiency: clinical and laboratory responses to therapy with transfer factor, Proc. Nat. Acad. Sci. U.S.A. 67:821, 1970.

Levine, B. B., Stember, R. H., and Fotino, M.: Ragweed hay fever: genetic control and linkage to HL-A haplotypes, Science 178:1201, 1972.

Lim, S.-D., *et al.*: Thymus-dependent lymphocytes of peripheral blood in leprosy patients, Infect. Immun. 9:394, 1974.

Lin, P. S., Cooper, A. G., and Wortis, H. H.: Scanning electron microscopy of human T-cell and B-cell rosettes, N. Engl. J. Med. 289:548, 1973.

Marsh, D. G., *et al.*: Association of the HL-A7 cross-reacting group with a specific reaginic antibody response in allergic man, Science 179:691, 1973.

McKay, E., and Thom, H.: Observations on neonatal tears, J. Pediatr. 75:1245, 1969.

Miller, J. F. A. P., *et al.*: Interaction between lymphocytes in immune responses, Cell. Immunol. 2:469, 1971.

Miller, L., Gitlin, D., and Hirvonen, T.: Pediatric progress, Hospital Tribune, April 23, 1973.

Mitchell, G. F., *et al.*: Immunological memory in mice. III. Memory to heterologous erythrocytes in both T cell and B cell populations and requirement for T cells in expression of B cell memory. Evidence using immunoglobulin allotype and mouse alloantigen theta markers with congenic mice, J. Exp. Med. 135:165, 1972.

Mitchison, N. A.: The carrier effect in the secondary response to hapten-protein conjugates. I. Measurement of the effect with transferred cells and objections to local environment hypothesis, Eur. J. Immunol. 1:10, 1971.

Mitchison, N. A.: The carrier effect in the secondary response to hapten-protein conjugates. II. Cellular cooperation, Eur. J. Immunol. 1:18, 1971.

Modabber, F.: Antigen-binding cells of the thymus, Contemp. Top. Immunobiol. 2:207, 1973.

Paraskevas, F., Orr, K. B., and Lee, S.-T.: Cell surface-associated gamma globulins in lymphocytes. III. Changes of γ-globulin-carrying lymphocytes during primary response, J. Immunol. 109:1254, 1972.

Parish, C. R.: Suppression of antibody formation and concomitant enhancement of cell-mediated immunity by acetoacetylated derivatives of *Salmonella* flagellin, Ann. N. Y. Acad. Sci. 181:108, 1971.

Paterson, R., *et al.:* Mucocutaneous candidiasis, anergy and a plasma inhibitor of cellular immunity: Reversal after amphotericin B therapy, Clin. Exp. Immunol. 9:595, 1971.

Pincus, S., Bianco, C., and Nussenzweig, V.: Increased proportion of complement-receptor lymphocytes in the peripheral blood of patients with chronic lymphocytic leukemia, Blood XL:303, 1972.

Preud'homme, J. L., and Seligmann, M.: Primary immunodeficiency with increased numbers of circulating B lymphocytes contrasting with hypogammaglobulinaemia, Lancet 1:442, 1972.

Raff, M. C.: Role of thymus-derived lymphocytes in the secondary humoral response in mice, Nature (Lond.) 226:1257, 1970.

Raff, M. C.: T and B lymphocytes and immune responses, Nature New Biol. 242:19, 1973.

Raff, M. C., and DePetris, S.: Movement of lymphocyte surface antigens and receptors: the fluid nature of the lymphocyte plasma membrane and its immunological significance, Fed. Proc. 32:48, 1973.

Rowe, D. S., *et al.:* IgD on the surface of peripheral blood lymphocytes of the human newborn, Nature New Biol. 242:155, 1973.

Sbarra, A. J., *et al.*: Role of the phagocyte in host-parasite interactions. XXXVIII. Metabolic activities of the phagocyte as related to antimicrobial action, J. Reticuloendothel. Soc. 12:109, 1972.

Schulkind, M. L., *et al.*: Transfer factor in the treatment of a case of chronic mucocutaneous candidiasis, Cell. Immunol. 3:606, 1972.

Siltzbach, L. E.: Sarcoidosis, in Samter, M. (ed.): *Immunological Diseases,* Vol. I. (2nd ed.; Boston: Little, Brown and Co., 1971).

Smith, R. T., Good, R. A., and Miescher, P. A. (eds.): *Ontogeny of Immunity* (Gainesville, Fla.: University of Florida Press, 1967).

Smith, R. T., Miescher, P. A., and Good, R. A. (eds.): *Phylogeny of Immunity* (Gainesville, Fla.: University of Florida Press, 1966).

Soothill, J. F., *et al.:* Some relationships between serum immunoglobulin deficiencies and infection in utero and in the early weeks of life, J. Pediatr. 75:1257, 1969.

Spitler, L. E., Levin, A. S., and Fudenberg, H. H.: Agammaglobulinemia, absent delayed hypersensitivity and lymphopenia without infection, Am. J. Med. 54:371, 1973.

Stein, H., Lennert, K., and Parwaresch, M. R.: Malignant lymphomas of B-cell type, Lancet 2:855, 1972.

Stjernswärd, J., *et al.*: Lymphopenia and change in distribution of human B and T lymphocytes in peripheral blood induced by irradiation for mammary carcinoma, Lancet 1:1352, 1972.

Strober, S., and Dilley, J.: Biological characteristics of T and B memory lymphocytes in the rat, J. Exp. Med. 137:1275, 1973.

Trainin, N., and Small, M.: Thymic humor factors, Contemp. Top. Immunobiol. 2:321, 1973.

Turk, J. L., and Bryceson, A. D. M.: Immunological phenomenon in leprosy and related diseases, Adv. Immunol. 13:209, 1971.

Uhr, J. W., Dancis, J., and Neuman, G. C.: Delayed hypersensitivity in premature neonatal humans, Nature (Lond.) 187:1130, 1960.

Uhr, J. W., et al.: The antibody response to bacteriophage φ X 174 in newborn premature infants, J. Clin. Invest. 41:1509, 1962.

Watson, J.: The role of humoral factors in the initiation of in vitro primary immune responses. III. Characterization of factors that replace thymus-derived cells, J. Immunol. 111:1301, 1974.

Weigle, W. O.: Immunological unresponsiveness, Adv. Immunol. 16:61, 1973.

Wheelock, E. F., Toy, S. T., and Stjernholm, R. L.: Interaction of viruses with human lymphocytes, in Amos, B. (ed.): *Progress in Immunology I* (New York: Academic Press, 1971), p. 787.

Williams, R. C., Jr., et al.: Studies of T- and B-lymphocytes in patients with connective tissue diseases, J. Clin, Invest. 52:283, 1973.

Wybran, J., Chantler, S., and Fudenberg, H. H.: Isolation of normal T cells in chronic lymphatic leukemia, Lancet 1:126, 1973.

Wybran, J., Levin, A. S., Spitler, L. E., and Fudenberg, H. H.: Rosette-forming cells, immunological deficiency diseases and transfer factor, N. Engl. J. Med. 288:710, 1973.

8 / Host-Parasite Interactions and Protective Host Immunity

LOCALIZATION AND PERSISTENCE OF MICROORGANISMS WITHIN THE HOST

Microorganisms may persist in host tissues for varying reasons (Table 8–1). Certain infectious agents produce localized infections and may not induce immune responses. It is intriguing that the two most prevalent venereal diseases seem not to induce specific long-lasting antimicrobial immunity. After effective treatments, second infections of syphilis and gonorrhea are common. As yet, the mode of pathogenesis of the syphilis spirochete has eluded investigators since the spirochetal form is identifiable only in the primary chancre and in the early secondary skin lesions. Are syphilis spirochetes or their products immunosuppressive? Do altered morphologic forms of the spirochete escape detection, but allow the disease to progress in untreated patients?

It has been argued that the gonococcus (*Neisseria gonorrhoeae*) primarily induces a localized infection in the urogenital tract and, therefore, does not adequately stimulate immune responses. This, too, is difficult to accept since the human host does mount an inflammatory response against the gonococcus and the microorganism is capable of invading the blood stream inducing septicemia, meningitis, osteomyelitis, arthritis and endocarditis. In the presence of antibiotics which inhibit cell wall synthesis, e.g., penicillin, the gonococcus can give rise to L forms (viable bacteria minus cell wall). Does this often occur in vivo under the influence of other inducers of L forms (e.g., high amino acid concentrations)? Also, the gonococcus, like the meningococcus, contains an endotoxin. Is the endotoxin responsible for the destruction of host phagocytes and is it immunosuppressive at the time bacterial antigens are released in lymphoid organs? Both the meningococcus and the gonococcus reside naturally only in man and do not survive outside the body. They require rather rich media and exacting cultural conditions for growth. Even though meningococci are carried as

TABLE 8-1.—LOCALIZATION OF MICROORGANISMS WITHIN THE HOST

1. Localized infection; abscess formation
2. Altered microbial surfaces presented to the host
   a. L forms of bacteria
   b. Borrelia species
   c. Protozoan pathogens
   d. Certain fungi (*Cryptococcus neoformans*)
3. Intracellular parasitisms
   a. Obligate intracellular parasites: all viruses and
      Chlamydia species and most rickettsia
   b. Facultative intracellular parasites
      (1) Within host macrophages (reticuloendothelial system)
         (a) Bacteria
            1) *Mycobacterium tuberculosis*
            2) All Brucella species
            3) *Salmonella typhosa* and certain other salmonellae
            4) *Francisella tularensis*
            5) *Listeria monocytogenes*
         (b) Certain protozoa, (e.g., *Toxoplasma gondii*)
         (c) Certain fungi, (e.g., *Cryptococcus neoformans, Histoplasma capsulatum*)
      (2) Within polymorphonuclear neutrophils
         (a) *Staphylococcus aureus* (only in some instances)
      (3) Within fibroblasts and macrophages
         (a) *Mycobacterium leprae*
      (4) Within or attached to cells of mucous membranes?
         (a) *Mycoplasma* species

microflora in the nasopharynx of some individuals, they are deadly pathogens when relocated within the host. In the absence of inflammation no systemic stimulation of the immune response occurs but it is possible that on the mucous membrane surfaces local production of IgA occurs. The secretory antibody may then enhance the phagocytosis of certain numbers of the microflora. *Neisseria meningitidis* is further subdued by competing with other nasopharyngeal flora for space and nutrients. Definitive answers to these problems are still being sought. An apparent paradox concerning the immune response to uncomplicated gonococcal urethritis has been reported. Antigonococcal reactivities (urethral secretory IgA, serum antibody and sensitized peripheral blood lymphocytes) were present in 13 of 24 males with multiple gonococcal infections. Do such observations suggest an inadequate protective immune response on the part of the host or do they imply that different antigenic strains of virulent gonococci exist as do meningococci?

Staphylococcus aureus tends to induce abscess formation in infected humans. The fibrin deposit demarcating the abscess functions as an osmotic barrier and restrains the entrance of immunoglobulins into the focus of infection. Certain virulent staphylococci excrete substances which are leukocidal and kill phagocytic cells. In some instances, viable staphylococci have been observed residing within the short-lived PMN's. Staphylococcal coagulase causes the deposition of fibrin around each coccus and thereby affords it a protective coating, for a time, within the phagocytic vacuole. First the fibrin must be digested away before the bacterium is attacked. Highly virulent staphylococci are equipped with a variety of substances to impair the host defense system but do not seem to possess a single "main virulence factor" against which protective host immunity may be mobilized. Recurrent osteomyelitis of prolonged duration has been induced by *S. aureus.* This microorganism can also undergo transition to L forms in the presence of antibiotics such as penicillin and re-emerge in full virulence after the antibiotic treatment ceases. Moreover, drug resistances as well as enterotoxigenicity (responsible for staphylococcal food poisoning) may be acquired by the staphylococci via bacterial genetic exchange mechanisms. The problems associated with staphylococcal infections in the human seem insoluble through immunologic means alone.

For the most part, staphylococci as well as pathogenic streptococci (beta hemolytic, group A *S. pyogenes*) and pneumococci are extracellular pyogenic bacterial pathogens which induce inflammatory responses and fever in the infected host. The main feature of protective host immunity in these infections appears to be antibody which binds to bacterial surface structures (the capsule of the pneumococcus, the M protein of the streptococcal cell wall). The antibody "roughs-up" the smooth bacterial surface making the surface sticky and thereby much easier for the phagocyte to ingest. Such antibodies are termed *immune opsonins.* Complement components via the alternate complement pathway may bind to the pneumococcal capsular carbohydrate and act as additional opsonizing factors.

In special circumstances, microorganisms may present the host defense systems with an altered or new surface. The significance of L forms in vivo is still speculative. The L form lacking a cell wall can be induced in the laboratory in a variety of manners: 3% glycine, soft agar and anaerobiosis; penicillin; high salt concentration and even antigen-antibody complexes. L forms of a number of gram-positive and gram-negative pathogenic bacteria have been found in infected humans and animals but always in the presence of the vegetative form of the same bacterium. The L forms are more sluggish metabolically than are the parent bacteria and, naturally, are resistant to antibiotics which impair cell wall synthesis. The main threat of L forms in vivo is the apparent re-emergence of infectious disease following the reversion of

L forms to the fully virulent parent form of the bacteria. *Borrelia recurrentis* is a vector-borne bacterial spirochete causing relapsing fever in man. This agent apparently induces a febrile disease followed by an afebrile period in which the surviving bacteria display new antigens; then a shorter febrile period ensues. A patient may exhibit three or four such relapses between febrile and afebrile periods. After a particular antigenic type has appeared and antibodies are made to it, it disappears from the blood. This versatile parasite apparently undergoes this "antigenic changing of coats" in vivo. Protozoan pathogens such as the malarial parasites can undergo their asexual life cycle in the human, displaying many different forms within liver parenchymal cells and human erythrocytes. Thus, it is difficult for the host immune system to ever get ahead of such parasites during infection. Certain saprophytes in nature such as the fungus *Cryptococcus neoformans,* display little, if any, capsule when isolated from soil. However, once the human is systemically infected, the cryptococcus, a facultative intracellular parasite of reticuloendothelial macrophages, may display a completely new and large chitinous-like capsule for which the host has no degradative enzymes.

All viruses, all chlamydia and most rickettsia* are obligate intracellular parasites. Viruses are molecular parasites containing either DNA or RNA. The nucleic acid supplies them with the necessary genetic information to usurp the host cell's synthetic machinery to replicate themselves or to become associated with the host cell's genetic material. Surface structures of viruses recognize susceptible host cells which contain receptor areas to which the viruses attach. Viruses are then taken up by the host cells by viropexis (pinocytosis). In general, immune responses involving both antibody and T cell responses directed against surface antigens of virus particles provide effective protective host immunity. Adequate immune responses can be made against chlamydia and rickettsia, which are now known to be bacteria with gram-negative type cell walls. Antibody to surface structures of these two groups of bacteria is presumed to be the main aspect of protective host immunity. However, the T cell-mediated immunities have yet to be assessed in infections by chlamydia and rickettsia. The agent responsible for inducing Reiter's syndrome (a triad consisting of conjunctivitis, nonbacterial urethritis and arthritis) may be a chlamydia. The microbial parasites considered facultative intracellular parasites of the reticuloendothelial macrophage are listed in Table 8–1.

R. quintana, causative agent of trench fever, can grow on enriched cell-free media and appears to have different permeability properties than other rickettsia.

These parasites are able to resist destruction within macrophages. It has been suggested that all of these parasites contain high amounts of structural lipid which may protect them from phagocytic digestion within the phagolysosome (secondary lysosome). Some of these parasites may stay within either the phagosome or phagolysosome after ingestion. Those which require chelation may multiply within the phagolysosome because chelation is favored at acid pH (the pH of the phagolysosome is approximately 5.5). Some facultative intracellular parasites are able to leave the secondary lysosome in a viable state and reside in the cytoplasm. Little is known of the method of egress into the cytoplasm. An unusual type of lecithinase has been associated with the ability of *Listeria monocytogenes* to enter the cytoplasm from the phagolysosome. The cytoplasmic compartment has a pH of approximately 7.0–7.2 and all of the necessary substances for intermediary metabolism. Thus, the facultative intracellular parasites are harbored in a favorable environment sheltered from the influence of antibody. Eventually, they exhaust the hospitality of the host cell through their multiplication, the host cell dies and they must search for new intracellular environments.

The most significant aspect of protective host immunity against the facultative intracellular parasites is cell-mediated immunity in which T cell and microbial antigen interactions release lymphokines, one of which is macrophage activation factor. This substance stimulates macrophages to heightened microbicidal activity. Instead of finding a hospitable environment within macrophages, these parasites find a lethally hostile environment within the activated cells. Only the induction of lymphokines is antigen-specific. Once activated, the macrophage is not selective as to which parasite it kills and degrades. However, macrophage cytophilic antibodies may act as opsonins to aid the ingestion of these parasites. Thus, activated macrophages to which cytophilic antibody is attached selectively ingest the parasite against which the antibody is directed.

M. leprae may be present in modified monocytes (lepra cells). This particular parasite still confronts us with many unsolved problems concerning its pathogenesis. Between contact and initial lesions, many years may pass. Incubation times of from a few months to 30 years have been observed for this agent. The microorganism must travel from the initial skin site via the bloodstream to other sites within the body, although it seems unable to multiply in the blood. Most lesions are associated with the skin and may be seen also in the nasopharynx, ears and mouth. Curiously, the peripheral nerves also exhibit lesions. Fibroblasts and monocytes contain leprosy bacilli, both in the bacillary (rod) form as well as round forms (L forms). As discussed in Chapter 7, humans with lepromatous leprosy contain macrophages teeming with leprosy bacilli. In leprosy, the cell-mediated immune mechanism of activating macrophages apparently is the mechanism of protective host resistance. Leprosy bacilli have never yet been successfully cultured in human cells in tissue culture. Yet, human leprosy bacilli have been cultivated in mouse foot pads. From these latter studies, the generation time of the bacillus was 20–30 days. The fact that humans are highly resistant to experimental infection by leprosy bacilli isolated from human lesions may be tentatively explained. Activated macrophages are not selective as to which parasites they destroy, thus they may be activated by any number of cell-mediated reactions against a variety of microbial parasites. Since the generation time of the leprosy bacillus is approximately 20–30 days, a likely possibility exists that during that time either (1) the macrophages containing leprosy bacilli will be activated or (2) that the initial monocytes might die liberating the leprosy bacilli which may then be taken up by activated monocytes. Further speculation might predict that tuberculoid leprosy would develop in those individuals whose immune systems are functionally intact but whose leprosy-containing monocytes accidentally missed being activated. However, the lepromatous form of disease may develop in individuals who are immunosuppressed by severe malnutrition or temporarily by a viral disease.

The mycoplasma are bacteria, lacking cell walls, whose "single cell" or minimum reproductive unit is the size of certain viral agents. The only established human pathogen among the mycoplasma is *M. pneumoniae,* which causes a primary atypical pneumonia. Other species of mycoplasma are present on the mucous membranes of the human. Although attempts to incriminate them in human disease are many, the same mycoplasma strains can always be found on the mucous membranes of healthy humans. Mycoplasma readily attach to sialic acid residues in the cell membrane. Apparently, these agents can live both intracellularly and extracellularly, tightly attached to the mammalian cell membrane. Pathogenic mycoplasma are fastidious in their growth requirements and exhibit the unusual need for sterols. Specific antibody can inhibit mycoplasmal reproduction. Antibody appears to be the main feature of protective host immunity against *M. pneumoniae.* Inactivated *M. pneumoniae* vaccines are effective in protecting some humans against either natural or experimental infection, but not all of those vaccinated develop antibody and are protected. Attempts are in progress to prepare living attenuated *M. pneumoniae* vaccines. *M. pneumoniae* infections in man induce antibody responses to a heterogenetic (streptococcus MG) antigen as well as cold agglutinins (antibodies which agglutinate only in the cold) for human erythrocytes. Cold agglutinin formation occurs more frequently and in approximately two-thirds of the patients. Thus, the nonspecific cold agglutinin titer (titer of 32 or greater) is used as a diagnostic aid.

MICROBIAL VIRULENCE FACTORS

Microorganisms are able to exert virulence in a number of ways. *Clostridium perfringens,* whose main virulence factor is an exotoxin (alpha-toxin) which is a lecithinase, is equipped with a variety of other virulence factors: hyaluronidase, collagenase, streptolysin-like substance, etc. Streptolysins destroy mammalian cell lysosomes. There are currently five serotypes of *C. perfringens* (A, B, C, D and E) which produce severe toxemias in man and animals. The lecithinase activity in itself is adequately devastating to the host. Lysing all host cell membranes, it destroys red cells as well as tissue cells. Also, many other bacteria come equipped with a variety of virulence factors such as *S. aureus* and *S. pyogenes.*

A list of microbial virulence factors is presented in Table 8–2. Antiphagocytic factors are usually a constitutive part of the microorganisms (e.g., pneumococcal capsules and M proteins of streptococcal cell walls). They cause a repulsion or negative chemotaxis of host phagocytes. Endotoxins which are a part of the membrane-cell wall complex of gram-negative bacteria and certain exotoxins (e.g., staphylococcal leukocidin), are antiphagocytic in that they kill cells, especially phagocytic cells. Endotoxins are not only directly toxic to phagocytes but to all cells of the reticuloendothelial system.

The bacterial exotoxins are mainly proteins secreted into the environment surrounding the bacteria. They act at specific sites in host cell metabolic processes. As examples: diphtheria toxin interferes with protein synthesis of the cells of susceptible mammalian hosts by

TABLE 8-2.—Mechanisms of Microbial Virulence and Host Alteration

1. Antiphagocytic factors
2. Endotoxins
3. Exotoxins
4. Enzymes and other factors
5. Intracellular parasitisms: obligate and facultative
6. Delayed hypersensitivity
7. Immune response to heterogenetic microbial antigens
8. Competition with host for nutrients

specifically inactivating translocation factor, T_2, of eucaryotic cells; the murine plague toxin interferes with the electron transport of the cytochrome system probably at the level of cytochrome Q reductase; tetanus toxin appears as a potent neurotoxin acting on the synthesis and liberation of acetylcholine. There are six antigenically distinct types (A, B, C, D, E and F) of botulinum toxin; type A (15,000 times more toxic than the most toxic drug known, aconitine) and type B botulinum toxin interfere with the release but not the synthesis of acetylcholine while type E toxin exerts less effect on the nerves and more severe gastrointestinal symptoms. The pathogenic mycoplasma can produce an exotoxin which is not protein but a toxic peroxide. Other than lecithinase, most microbial enzymes elaborated by pathogenic bacteria are not the main bacterial virulence factors, although they may contribute to the maintenance of the bacteria in host tissues. As previously cited, coagulase, either bound to the staphylococci or free, functions to temporarily protect the staphylococci from digestion within phagocytic vacuoles. Hyaluronidase which depolymerizes hyaluronic acid is elaborated by certain pathogenic streptococci, staphylococci and *C. perfringens.*

Enzymes which induce the digestion of fibrinogen and the lysis of fibrin clots have been called fibrinolysins or streptokinases when elaborated by most strains of hemolytic streptococci of group A, and by some strains of groups C and G. Staphylokinase elaborated by *S. aureus* can even be observed to lyse the clots formed by coagulase by activating plasminogen to plasmin (fibrinolytic enzyme).

Group A streptococci elaborate streptolysin O (antigenic and inactivated by oxygen) and streptolysin S (not antigenic). Antistreptolysin is used to diagnose and follow the course of streptococcal infections. The streptolysins appear to lyse red cells only in vitro. The cytolytic action of streptolysin in tissue cells is mediated through the release of the cell's lysosomal enzymes which may occur in vivo. Antigenically, streptolysin O is related to the oxygen labile pneumolysin elaborated by pneumococci, the tetanolysin of *C. tetani* and a similar factor from *C. perfringens.* Certain streptococci and some staphylococci elaborate an NADase which exerts leukotoxicity via enzymatic action on the NAD substrate. A variety of other enzymes (collagenase, proteases, amylases, nucleases, etc.) are elaborated by bacteria.

Investigations concerning virulence factors of dermatophytes (fungi which parasitize the skin) have yielded little knowledge of their mechanisms of parasitism other than the fact that they elaborate keratolytic factors. Dissolution and utilization of keratin may be sufficient for dermatophytes to successfully parasitize skin.

As has been discussed, both obligate and facultative intracellular parasitisms represent an advantage to the microorganism in the unimmunized host. Both antibody and cell-mediated immunity responses are induced as host defense mechanisms against these parasites. Of the two responses, the cell-mediated immune mechanism of macrophage activation is more significant in host defense against the facultative intracellular parasites and in certain viral diseases. The interaction of sensitized T lymphocytes with microbial antigen and possibly with microbially altered host antigens in vivo may cause extensive elaboration of lymphokines. Even though this same mechanism is held responsible for ridding the tissues of these parasites at the cellular level, certain of the lymphokines may injure other host cells and contribute to granuloma formation, i.e., manifestation of delayed hypersensitivity. It is possible that more lymphotoxic factors are elaborated as a result of certain T cell-antigen interactions.

In some individuals, an unfortunate byproduct of the immune response to certain bacterial antigens is the formation of antibody which cross-reacts with human tissue antigens, i.e., heterogenetic antigens. The formation of such antibody stimulated by a heterogenetic antigen has been offered as an explanation for poststreptococcal sequelae, i.e., the generation of rheumatic fever and poststreptococcal glomerulonephritis. Similar explanations have been used to explain the genesis of ulcerative colitis (*E. coli* shares antigenicity with the intestinal mucosa). Also, antibodies reacting with allografts have been observed in guinea pigs, rabbits, mice, rats and dogs following immunization with a variety of bacteria (*S. aureus, S. epidermidis,* and *S. pyogenes*).

In reality, all microbial parasites compete with the host for nutrients or substances used in their replication. However, little definitive information exists concerning the contribution of other microorganisms to the pathogenesis by a given parasite, as seen in microbial synergisms such as fusospirochetal disease. Associated bacterial cells seem important in supplying essential nutrients to the protozoan *Entamoeba histolytica.* Under certain circumstances, cultures of mixed bacterial intestinal flora have been shown to increase the invasiveness and infectivity of *E. histolytica.*

PROTECTIVE HOST IMMUNITY

Antibody-mediated protective immunity may be characterized as one or more of the following. (1) Antibodies which react with surface structures (capsule, cell wall) of a microorganism enhance phagocytic ingestion and are called *immune opsonins.* Immune opsonins play a significant role in protective host resistance against pneumococcal and streptococcal infections. (2) Antibodies which bind to "soluble" antigens and thereby prevent either toxic action (of bacterial exotoxins) or infection of host cells by viral particles are called *neutralizing antibodies.* (3) The only microorganisms whose reproduction is inhibited by antibody are two groups of bacteria, the cell wall-less mycoplasma and the spirochetal leptospires. In the case of the mycoplasma this antibody may be directed against protein surface antigens. Such antibody activity may be referred to as *multiplication-inhibiting antibody.* (4) Although bacteriolysis of certain gram-negative bacteria by *bacteriolytic antibody* and complement is readily demonstrated in vitro, the efficacy of such action in vivo may be questioned. First, gram-negative bacteriolysis possibly contributes to endotoxicity and endotoxin shock (see Chapter 4). In the treatment of brucellosis patients receiving high doses of antibiotics that may penetrate reticulo-endothelial macrophages (e.g., streptomycin), fatal endotoxin-like shock may ensue when liberated dead bacteria react with antibody and complement in the circulation. Consequently, treatment of such patients involves the carefully monitored use of antibiotics and steroids. Second, the gram-negative microflora residing on mucous membrane surfaces, such as *E. coli* in the gut, will more likely be controlled by secretory IgA acting as an *opsonin.* Third, if any complement-fixing IgM or IgG would become involved in bacteriolysis of gram-negative bacterial flora in the gut, the reaction would probably be minimal and thereby limit damage.

Toxicity of bacterial endotoxins is attributed to the lipid constituent. However, isolated lipid (lipid A) is not nearly as toxic as is the intact lipopolysaccharide. Lipid A as it exists in the naturally occurring lipopolysaccharide (endotoxin, O antigen) moiety or bound to various serum albumin carrier molecules appears more toxic in rabbits than is lipid A alone. *Endotoxin tolerance* or "pyrogenic tolerance" is a phenomenon in which resistance to the pyrogenic and lethal effects of endotoxin can be imparted to rabbits for a period of time following repeated injections of small but increasing amounts of endotoxin. Rabbits can also be protected against endotoxic pyrogenicity following injections of increasing increments of lipid A conjugated to either human or bovine serum albumin. There is some indication that anti-O antibody, directed essentially against the carbohydrate portion of endotoxin, is involved in the late phase of endotoxin tolerance in the rabbit. These same antibodies (anti-O) may be involved in endotoxin shock (see Chapter 4). At present, neither endotoxin shock nor endotoxin tolerance is understood. Whether endotoxin tolerance plays a role in resistance of humans to endogenous gram-negative microflora is uncertain.

Inducible nonimmunologic factors may contribute to protective host immunity during certain infectious processes. *Interferon* is a protein-aceous substance induced locally in the human and animal host in response to infections by many viruses and other obligate intracellular parasites (rickettsia and chlamydia) as well as by facultative intracellular parasites. It may also be released as a lymphokine by activated T cells. Interferon exhibits an antiviral effect early (first 3 to 4 days) in a viral infection, after which the host cells appear refractory to its action for a short time (5 days). In some manner, interferon protects susceptible host cells from translating viral-coded messages, yet does not interfere with the cell's inherent translation of messages into host cell proteins. Generally, interferon is not inducer-specific as are immune responses but is host species-specific; i.e., human interferon best protects human cells and not chicken cells and vice versa. Polyanions (such as double-stranded reovirus RNA, the double-stranded replicating viral RNA's of single-stranded RNA viruses, synthetic polynucleotides, synthetic polycarboxylic acids, pyran copolymers, and bacterial endotoxins) all can stimulate interferon formation and/or release from host cells. *Ablastin* is another host-produced nonimmunologic factor which functions in host protection against certain protozoan parasites, e.g., trypanosomes. It apparently acts by interfering with the nucleic acid and protein synthetic pathways of the trypanosomes. Consequently, these parasites are prevented from multiplying and the host is afforded the opportunity to mobilize more effective immunologic intervention.

Specific cell-mediated immunity, the result of sensitized T cells reacting with either specific microbial antigens or microbe-altered host antigens, has only been actively studied in recent years. The release of lymphokines with the ensuing entrapment and activation of macrophages may well be the more significant immune reactivity in host protection against all the facultative intracellular parasites and many, if not most, of the viral pathogens. The role of antibody to surface antigens as the main aspect of protective host immunity in tuberculosis, typhoid fever, salmonellosis, brucellosis, tularemia, etc., has been questioned for years. Yet these antibodies may act as opsonins and even may exist as cytophilic antibodies on macrophages. Thus, they may exert the cooperative effect of opsonization of these parasites by macrophages, which, in turn, are activated by a lymphokine to heightened microbicidal activity. The role of neutralizing antibody as the main host defense against viral disease has been so entrenched in our thinking that it has taken the observations of rather bizarre clinical conditions to stimulate a reconsideration of host protection against viral parasites. The most compelling observations have come from children with deficient cell-mediated immune potential following vaccination with vaccinia viruses. These children displayed high titers of viral neutralizing antibodies yet suffered progressive vaccina disease. Reversal of this condition was accomplished only after reconstitution of specific T cell immunity (dialyzable transfer factors prepared from lymphoid populations rich in T cells from immune individuals).

Recent evidence indicates that cell-mediated immunity is raised against influenza virus. Let us consider a highly speculative set of events that *just may occur* in the nonimmune but normally immunocompetent human. Bear in mind that the response to influenza virus involves the production of secretory IgA, serum IgG, IgM and IgA antibodies, and cell-mediated immunity. Upon entry into the nasopharynx, the virus particles enter cells of the respiratory mucosa. Within 12 to 24 hours interferon is released by the infected cells which should protect, to some degree, uninfected cells from being parasitized by virus for 3–4 days. At this same time, newly synthesized viral particles start being released. During the initial days of the infection local IgA and, perhaps, local T cell responses are being induced. As the completed influenza virus particles are pinched off the infected cells' membranes and spewed into the microenvironment, some may parasitize uninfected and unprotected host cells, some may be disseminated to induce systemic antibody (serum IgM, IgG and IgA) responses, others may be neutralized by local secretory antibody and disposed of within phagocytes, while others may interact with virus-specific T cells which release lymphokines. Among the lymphokines is interferon. Thus, a reinforcement of the interferon protection occurs. Also, macrophages are trapped and activated, thereby enhancing the phagocytic mechanism. Antibody-bound (opsonized) virus may be more readily ingested and digested. Inflammatory host responses are more usual in bacterial invasion but are not seen in early virus infections. Eventually, the virus infection is contained by these cooperative processes (immune and nonimmune) and the virus is eradicated from the infected host. By the time that significant titers of antibody are present in the serum, the infectious process has been quelled.

Of all the virus parasites, the influenza viral antigens are best defined. The outermost surface of the influenza virus particles exposed to the host consists of a lipoprotein nucleocapsid to which hemagglutinin and neuraminidase glycoprotein spikes are attached. There are approximately 5 times as many hemagglutinin spikes as there are neuraminidase spikes. The major protective antibody responses are directed against these types of spikes. Assays of viral neutralization by antibody are usually performed by observing the neutralization of infectivity in vitro. The inhibition of viral cytopathologic effects on susceptible cell cultures is observed. Measures of antibody include the hemagglutination-inhibition assay where specific antibody bound to hemagglutinin spikes prevents viral attachment to erythrocyte receptors and thereby prevents the formation of hemagglutination patterns. Neuraminidase inhibition may also be assayed since neuraminidase action appears responsible for elution of virus from erythrocytes (following hydrolysis of galactose-N-acetylneuraminic acid bonds). Symptoms of disease appear within 24–48 hours after exposure to virus with clinical illness apparent for about 6–7 days during which time virus may be shed to other individuals. Secondary bacterial infections usually occur 5–10 days after exposure to virus. High titers of antiviral antibody are present in the serum within 2–3 weeks after initiation of infection. The epidemiology of influenza virus is uniquely associated with the hemagglutinin and neuraminidase antigens. The three types (A, B and C) of influenza virus are identified serologically by their own type-specific nucleocapsid antigen. The A strains are the only influenza viruses which have designated nucleocapsid subtypes (A_0, A_1, A_2). The nucleocapsid antigen is called the S, for soluble antigen, while the hemagglutinin (H) and neuraminidase (N) antigens are together called V antigens since they are envelope antigens associated with the viral particle. In both H and N antigens, genetically determined alterations can occur. These changes are responsible for the emergence of epidemics of "new" influenza strains among the A type influenza viruses. Both major and minor alterations of either or both of these V antigens may and have occurred. When a major change occurs, no cross-immunity exists and pandemics occur easily. Such change in a virus is called a major *antigenic shift* and involves major antigenic alterations of H and N antigens. A minor change in one or both of the V antigens is called an *antigenic drift.*

Because influenza A viruses are present in some animal species (birds, horses and swine), it has been suggested that these animal reservoirs may serve as a source of new epidemic viral strains. This theory may also explain the reemergence in the human host of an influenza strain that was present in humans many years previously. Although antigenic differences in influenza B viruses exist between strains, these differences are slight and therefore the S antigens are not designated as subtypes. To date, only one type of influenza C virus is documented.

Agammaglobulinemic children recover normally from many viral infections while children with deficits in cell-mediated immune potential show poor recovery from certain viral agents. In immunologically competent individuals, Dulbecco and Ginsberg have observed that viruses which cause viremias tend to stimulate long-lasting immunity in which circulating antibody persists, e.g., measles or mumps virus; most, but not all, viruses which exhibit acute localized infections do not seem to stimulate protection against second infections, e.g., influenza viruses. However, the role of secretory IgA antibodies against respiratory viruses is critical. For example, the initial infection of a child with a parainfluenza virus is often severe, while adults infected with the same virus are usually not seriously ill and exhibit no fever. Most adults examined have detectable serum antibodies to all types of parainfluenza virus yet little, if any, IgA antibody in their nasal secretions. However, detectable IgA antibodies are absent from nasal secretions within 1–6 months following infection. Dulbecco and Ginsberg suggest that adults experience less severe parainfluenza infections because they are able to mount quickly an effective secondary secretory antibody response. No definitive proof exists as an explanation for the fact that humans do display lasting immunity against some viral agents. Dulbecco and Ginsberg note that the viruses against which man shows long-lasting immunity are those which are ubiquitous in our environment, e.g., mumps, measles, poliomyelitis and chickenpox viruses. Thus, they may serve as repeated antigenic stimuli. Although never proved, it has been suggested that the persistence of latent viruses in the tissues provides the opportunity for periodic antigenic stimulation.

Both antibody, especially secretory IgA, and cell-mediated immunity play significant but separate roles in host resistance to viral parasitisms. Antibodies in serum and extracellular spaces undoubtedly function as neutralizing antibodies, as does secretory IgA in the mucous membranes. (Waldman and associates found a ratio of 2.5:1 of IgG:IgA in bronchioalveolar fluid of humans, while the IgG:IgA ratio in serum was 5:1 and in nasal secretions was 1:3.)

Cell-mediated immune resistance with subsequent macrophage activation may be of critical importance against viral agents that (1) disseminate contiguously from cell to cell and thereby are shielded from neutralization by antibody, and/or (2) alter the host cell surface so that it is no longer normal "self." Considering the large numbers of viral progeny replicated from one infected cell, it is not remarkable that both limbs of the immune response may be activated and necessary to rid the tissues of viral parasites. However, the host immune responses are not able to effect removal of a host cell in which a virus or its genetic information lies latent if the host cell surface antigens remain normal.

SUGGESTED READINGS

Coonrod, J. D.: Properdin levels in pneumonia, N. Engl. J. Med. 288:1302, 1973.

Davis, R. D., et al. (eds.): Microbiology (2nd ed.; Hagerstown, Md.: Harper and Row, Publishers, 1973).

Dulbecco, R., and Ginsberg, H. S.: in Davis, R. D., et al. (eds.): Microbiology (2nd ed.; Hagerstown, Md.: Harper & Row, Publishers, 1973).

Fowles, R. E., et al.: The enhancement of macrophage bacteriostasis by products of activated lymphocytes, J. Exp. Med. 138:952, 1973.

Ganguly, R.: Rubella immunization of volunteers via the respiratory tract, Infect. Immunol. 8:497, 1973.

Johnston, R. B., Jr., Newman, S. L., and Struth, A. G.: An abnormality of the alternate pathway of complement activation in sickle-cell disease, N. Engl. J. Med. 288:803, 1973.

Joklik, W. K., and Smith, D. T. (eds.): Zinsser Microbiology (15th ed.; New York: Appleton-Century-Crofts, 1972).

Kearns, D. H., et al.: Paradox of the immune response to uncomplicated gonococcal urethritis, N. Engl. J. Med. 289:1170, 1973.

Mackaness, G. B.: Delayed Hypersensitivity and the Mechanism of Cellular Resistance to Infection, in Amos, B. (ed.): Progress in Immunology I (New York: Academic Press, 1971), p. 413.

Mackaness, G. B.: The J. Burns Amberson Lecture—The induction and expression of cell-mediated hypersensitivity in the lung, Am. Rev. Resp. Dis. 101:813, 1971.

Smadel, J. E.: Intracellular infection and the carrier state, Science 140:153, 1963.

Suter, E., and Ramseier, H.: Cellular reactions in infection, Adv. Immunol. 4:117, 1964.

Trager, W.: Some aspects of intracellular parasitism, Science 183:269, 1974.

Waldman, R. H., Spencer, C. S., and Johnson, J. E., III: Respiratory and systemic cellular and humoral immune responses to influenza virus vaccine administered parenterally or by nose drops, Cell. Immunol. 3:294, 1972.

Wybran, J., and Fudenberg, H. H.: Thymus-derived rosette-forming cells in various human disease states: cancer, lymphoma, bacterial and viral infections, and other diseases, J. Clin. Invest. 52:1026, 1973.

Wybran, J., and Fudenberg, H. H.: Thymus-derived rosette-forming cells (Editorial), N. Engl. J. Med. 288:1072, 1973.

9 / Mechanisms of Immunologic Injury

The terms immunologic injury, clinical allergy and clinical hypersensitivity are synonymous, and are used to describe immunologically mediated injury. Gell and Coombs described four types of immunologic injury (types I–IV) to which Roitt added a fifth (type V).

TYPE I—ANAPHYLACTIC TYPE INJURY

Anaphylactic type immunologic injury is the same as that previously described as immediate type hypersensitivity. In the human species, this type of injury is primarily IgE-mediated, although in certain individuals IgG-mediated anaphylactic type injury has been observed. In atopic individuals, those who have inherited the predisposition to form IgE-type allergic responses, allergies to foods, drugs, insect venoms and inhalant antigens readily develop. Common inhalant allergenic substances include animal danders, feathers, pollens of grasses, weeds and trees, and house dust which includes fragments of dried mites. The term *allergen* is used to describe an antigen which induces the allergic state and subsequently provokes an allergic response.

The acute symptoms of serum sickness are attributed to IgE-mediated responses to foreign serum proteins, e.g., bovine or equine serum proteins. Since IgE binds preferentially to mast cells disseminated throughout the tissues, this type of antibody is described as capable of fixing to the skin (homocytotropic).

The immunologic events leading to anaphylactic type reactions are as follows. IgE molecules bound by the Fc region to mast cell membranes interact with the allergenic determinant of the antigen (Figs. 9–1 and 9–2). Apparently, this binding induces an allosteric conformational change in the membrane-bound IgE which then emits a signal to the membrane, which, in turn, signals the cell to degranulate, releasing histamine and other vasoactive substances. Roitt suggests that the first signal (IgE-mediated effect on the membrane) may

156

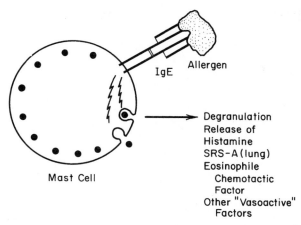

Fig. 9-1.—Mechanism of antigen-mediated release of the chemical mediators of anaphylaxis. Fc region of IgE molecule bound to mast cell membrane; antigen bound to Fab portions of antibody immunoglobulin.

well be adenyl cyclase. Within seconds to minutes after exposure to the specific allergen, a sensitized individual with anaphylactic type allergy will exhibit symptoms (hence the term immediate hypersensitivity). Extensive anaphylaxis may lead to respiratory collapse and death.

Orange and Austen have studied the mediators of anaphylactic reactions. (1) Histamine increases vascular permeability apparently by inducing a separation of the endothelial cells along their boundaries, exposing the basement membrane. Plasma readily leaks through the exposed membrane. Histamine also induces contraction of smooth muscle in the presence of calcium ions, and provokes pain and itching. In physiologic concentrations histamine activates adenyl cyclase and intracellular cyclic adenosine 3',5'-monophosphate (cAMP) accumulates in human peripheral white blood cells. As a consequence, IgE-mediated release of histamine from these cells is inhibited. (2) In several species including the human, slow reacting substance (SRS-A) is an acidic lipid with a molecular weight of 900 to 1,250. SRS-A is responsible for the bronchial spasms of asthmatics and induces contraction of human smooth muscle in vitro. Agents capable of increasing cAMP levels appear to inhibit the antigen-induced histamine release, while substances that effect a decrease in the intracellular levels of cAMP enhance the liberation of slow reacting substance (SRS-A). (3) Eosinophilic chemotactic factor of anaphylaxis (ECF-A), molecular weight of 500 to 1,000, specifically attracts eosinophils (Fig. 9–3). Eosinophilic cell infiltrates are characteristic of sites of

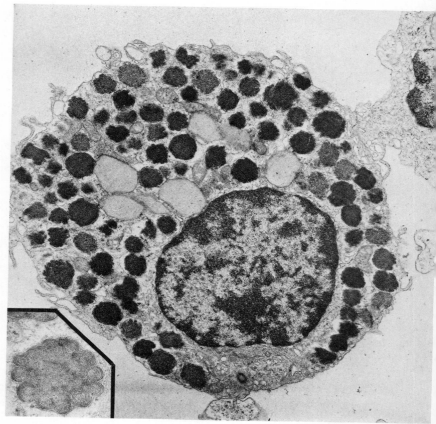

Fig. 9-2.—Electronmicrograph of mast cell showing single nucleus and cytoplasm filled with large membrane-bound electron-dense granules with a complex internal organization. *Inset,* high power electronmicrograph of a mast cell granule showing "scroll-like" internal organization.

immediate type hypersensitivity. (4) Serotonin (5-hydroxytryptamine), kallikrein and certain of the prostaglandins (for example, $PGF_{2\alpha}$) are also considered mediators of the anaphylactic type of tissue injury.

Several laboratory technics are used to demonstrate anaphylactic-type reactions with sera from atopic individuals or sensitized guinea pigs. (1) Anaphylactic shock may be induced in sensitized guinea pigs (sensitized to allergen, e.g., horse serum) following intravenous or intracardial injection of allergen. (2) Passive cutaneous anaphylaxis (PCA) involves the injection of high dilutions of serum containing

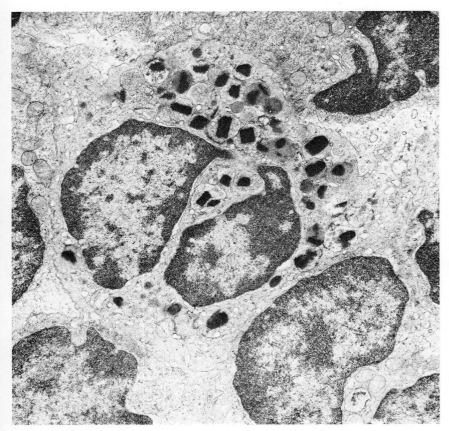

Fig. 9-3.—Electronmicrograph of eosinophilic granulocyte, showing a bi-lobed nucleus and numerous membrane-bound granules with dense internal crystalloid structures of various shapes and sizes.

either homocytotropic or heterocytotropic* antibody into the skin of an unsensitized animal, followed 3–17 hours later by an intravenous injection of antigen plus a dye (Evans blue). Because of the localized immunologic reaction, vasoactive substances are released resulting in increased capillary permeability and dissemination of the blue dye. (3) Human sera from atopic individuals can be injected into the skin of nonatopic volunteers followed 24 hours later by injection of specific

*Heterocytotropic antibody is a skin-fixing antibody from another species, e.g., human IgG or IgE into guinea pig. Homocytotropic antibody is a skin-fixing antibody from same species, e.g., guinea pig gamma₁ globulin into guinea pig.

allergen. An immediate wheal and flare inflammatory reaction (formation of a hive) develops within seconds to minutes after injection of the allergenic antigen. The site itches and may be painful. In patients with food allergies, hives may first develop after digestion begins, when allergenic substances are released into the circulation. Hives develop wherever allergen interacts with cell-bound IgE in the interstitial tissues. Also, local irritations to the gut mucosa may occur with subsequent symptomatology. (4) Sensitized human or animal sera containing cytotropic antibodies can be shown to induce degranulation of mast cells in vitro. (5) In the Schultz-Dale technic, strips of muscle from the uterus of a sensitized guinea pig are connected to a kymograph. Upon exposure to allergen, the muscle strips contract, mast cells degranulate and histamine and other substances are released. Using the same method, uterine muscle from an unsensitized animal may be passively sensitized with serum containing cytotropic antibody. Subsequent exposure to antigen induces the same type of response: contraction, histamine release, etc.

TYPE II—CYTOTOXIC TYPE INJURY

Cytotoxic injury to tissue cells may be antibody-mediated.

Immune Cytolysis of Erythrocytes

Immunologically mediated cytolysis of erythrocytes was unsatisfactorily explained for many years. Even though erythrophagocytosis, particularly by monocytes, may be seen in the peripheral blood of patients undergoing autoimmune hemolytic disease, phagocytosis as the sole mechanism of red cell destruction does not account for the massive and precipitous destruction of erythrocytes seen in certain of these patients with the warm-type antierythrocyte antibody. In vitro the warm-type autoantibody is usually unable to agglutinate or lyse human red cells even in the presence of complement at 37° C. Erythrocyte destruction by warm-type antibody is apparently not complement-dependent, although, in some individuals, activated complement components (C3 and C4) have been identified on the erythrocyte membrane.

Using the Coombs' test, Leddy and Swisher have described three patterns of direct antiglobulin reactions with washed erythrocytes from patients with autoimmune hemolytic disease. Certain red cells were found to have only IgG present on their membranes; others had both IgG and complement components, while still others had only complement components on their surfaces. In all antierythrocyte autoantibody populations studied, the IgG$_1$ subclass of immunoglobulin predominated. The preceding observations are the basis for the generalization that *warm-type immune cytolysis of erythrocytes is not necessarily complement-dependent and is usually mediated by IgG-type autoantibody.*

In many instances of acquired hemolytic anemia, the erythrocyte antigens against which autoantibody is directed are antigens of the Rh system other than $Rh_o(D)$. However, IgG autoantibodies of non-Rh specificity are usually associated with the in vivo binding of complement to the patient's red blood cells. In drug-induced hemolytic anemias the warm-type autoantibody is usually IgG, but a few instances have been reported in which other classes of immunoglobulins (IgM, IgA, and IgD) are involved in immune cytolysis in addition to the IgG class. In penicillin-induced hemolytic disease, the warm-type autoantibody is directed against only the penicillin which is passively adsorbed to the red cell surface. On the other hand, warm-type IgG autoantibody formed in patients with alpha-methyldopa-induced hemolytic disease appears to be a true autoantibody with specificity directed against erythrocyte antigens. In rare instances, red cells, white blood cells and platelets may be injured as a result of immune complex formation. Drugs best able to induce this type of hemolytic disease are quinine, quinidine and stibophen. The drug-antibody complex may bind complement at the surface of blood cells and platelets.

Certain drug-antibody combinations show a marked affinity for the membrane of red cells at which site complement is activated, even though the drug-antibody complex readily dissociates from the erythrocytes. In such instances, the Coombs' test is usually positive only for complement, while in penicillin-induced hemolytic anemias the patients' red cells are usually Coombs-positive only for IgG.

The mechanism of erythrocyte lysis is as follows. As depicted in Figure 9–4, the Fc region of the immunoglobulin is attached to receptors on mononuclear cells, mainly macrophages and possibly lymphocytes. The Fab portion of the antibody binds to red cell antigens. Since erythrocytes lack internal membrane structure the cell is sphered and, unable to withstand the forces of sphering, lyses. The remaining erythrocyte stroma is presumably phagocytized. It is not remarkable then that some of the antibody-coated red cells may be ingested by polymorphonuclear neutrophils or mononuclear phagocytes. Thus, the main mechanism of red cell destruction is erythrocyte fragmentation. Erythrophagocytosis may be seen in the reticulo-endothelial system of patients with autoimmune hemolytic anemia, e.g., in the macrophages of the spleen, liver, bone marrow and, occasionally, in lymph nodes. In the course of viral diseases such as

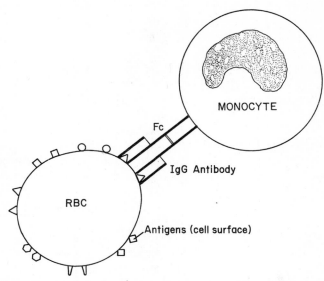

Fig. 9-4.—Sphering mechanism in immune cytolysis of red blood cells (*RBC*). Fab portions of antibody immunoglobulin bound to erythrocyte membrane antigens; *Fc* region of immunoglobulin attached to a mononuclear cell.

infectious mononucleosis in which hyperplasia of the reticuloendothelial and lymphatic systems is induced, autoimmune hemolytic disease with the warm-type autoantibody may occasionally occur.

Warm-type autoantibody-induced hemolytic disease may occur at all ages, although it is relatively rare in children. The incidence of this disease increases with age, with postmenopausal women being the usual victims. Autoimmune hemolytic disease may occur idiopathically or in combination with malignancies, e.g., chronic lymphocytic leukemia.

The attachment of the cold-type antierythrocyte autoantibody to the red cell requires colder temperatures, apparently to assume the necessary three-dimensional conformation. Cold agglutinins are mainly IgM immunoglobulins. These antibodies readily agglutinate red cells at 0–5° but are not able to do so at temperatures exceeding 30° C. Thus, in vivo, little opportunity exists for erythrocyte agglutination to occur. Yet, temperatures of 28–31° C may occur in the blood capillaries of exposed skin sites (nose, fingers, etc.) in cold weather. Presumably, cold-activated antibodies bind to red cells at these sites. Binding of complement is necessary for hemolysis to occur. For the IgM-complement-dependent immune cytolysis to be initiated, the patient must first be exposed to cold and then be returned to a warm environment, since the participation of the complement cascade occurs only at warmer temperatures (37° C). Consequently, acute intermittent massive hemolysis follows within minutes to hours after exposure to cold. The degree of chilling necessary to trigger hemolysis is highly variable from patient to patient. The combination of red cells, antibody and complement may lead to outright lysis of the erythrocyte; antibody with sublytic amounts of complement may cause sphering and red cell fragmentation as previously described. Even though the IgM class of immunoglobulins is the predominant cold-type antierythrocyte auto-antibody, cold-type antibodies have also been observed to be of the IgG class. The latter (IgG) antibodies are usually nonagglutinating in vitro but cause hemolysis in vivo. They are referred to as cold hemolysins and also activate complement.

Red cell antigens against which cold-type antierythrocyte antibodies develop are I, i, and P. In patients infected with *M. pneumoniae*, a transitory elevation in cold agglutinins of the IgM class, directed against the I red cell antigen, may occur. In patients with infectious mononucleosis, anti-i cold-reactive antierythrocyte antibodies of the IgG class may be found. In the cold hemolysin syndrome seen idiopathically, or in late syphilis (Jarisch-Herxheimer reaction) or transitorily in virus infections, the antigenic specificity of the autoantibody is usually anti-P. The sera of individuals with chronic cold agglutinin disease may contain an homogenous IgM spike of such magnitude upon electrophoresis that this disease may be confused with Waldenstöm's macroglobulinemia.

Antibody-Mediated Cytotoxicity of Other Cells

The binding of cytophilic IgM and IgG by their Fc regions to mononuclear cells (macrophages) may account for a significant degree of in vivo cytotoxicity directed against cells other than the erythrocyte. This type of reaction may well involve complement activation since complement receptors are also present on these mononuclear cells. Subsequent necrosis of the target cells occurs after the attachment of the Fab portions of the immunoglobulin molecules. The target cell may be any tissue cell displaying membrane antigens against which the antibody specificity is directed. Even though T cells are markedly cytotoxic in vitro, their capacities to destroy tumor cells and to mediate autoimmune injury in vivo are held in some doubt. Greenberg and associates cite evidence that antibody-mediated cytotoxic injury is caused by immunoglobulins bound by their Fc region to monocyte membranes. These monocytes were not phagocytically active at the time of identification. Such antibody-mediated cytotoxic reactions would be beneficial if the target cells were tumor cells but adverse if the target cells were allograft or normal tissue cells.

Free antibody in combination with complement is able to induce cytotoxic damage to cultured target cells. For example, sera from patients with Hashimoto's disease, an organ-specific autoimmune disease involving the thyroid, are cytotoxic for trypsin-dispersed cultured human thyroid cells in the presence of complement. Whether this mechanism functions in vivo in these patients is uncertain.

TYPE III—IMMUNE COMPLEX-MEDIATED INJURY

The generation of injurious complexes composed of antigen-antibody-complement can occur in vivo when high titers of complement-binding precipitating antibodies (IgM and IgG) are present in the circulation and when a source of specific, soluble antigen is available in the tissues. The generation of injurious immune complexes occurs in the presence of moderate antigen excess. (It has been argued that the formation of antigen-antibody complexes in the presence of great antigen excess would yield soluble noninjurious complexes. If antigen-antibody complexes formed in the presence of antibody excess, the resulting complexes would tend to be larger and insoluble and should be readily ingested by phagocytes and thus, also, noninjurious. However, it is difficult to extrapolate from in vitro observations to the dynamic in vivo situation.) Cochrane has shown that when soluble immune complexes reach the size of 19S molecules they tend to be injurious in that they settle out and stick to endothelial surfaces of blood vessels, glomeruli and even synovium. The complement cascade is activated and inflammatory mediators are released. Polymorphonuclear neutrophils are attracted and in their attempts to clear up the deposits, digest regions of the basement membrane, affording passage of blood cells and serum proteins into the tissues, urine or joints (Figs. 9–5 and 9–6).

The Arthus reaction and the chronic symptoms of serum sickness are examples of immune complex-mediated injury. In the local Arthus reaction, antigen is injected intradermally in an animal or individual with high titers of serum antibody. In the systemic Arthus reaction, antigen is injected into the tissues (e.g., intramuscularly) and diffuses out from the injection site toward capillaries and blood vessels. Both reactions are visible within 4–6 hours after antigen injection and are characterized by hemorrhagic necrosis. The skin site exhibits a central area of frank hemorrhage surrounded by erythema. The systemic reaction may be so severe that the hemorrhagic necrosis of the blood vasculature leads to shock and death. The outcome of a systemic Arthus reaction is usually evident by 24–36 hours after injection of antigen. Antigen diffuses into the blood vessels from the tissues and meets with antibody on the endothelial side of the blood vessel. Complement is activated, inflammation ensues, serum leaks into the tissues where more antigen-antibody complexes form and more complement activation occurs. Polymorphonuclear neutrophils attempt to clear the complexes and dead cells and in the process digest away more of the basement membrane of the blood vessel, causing hemorrhage into the tissue spaces. Roitt considers Farmer's lung disease as an intrapulmonary Arthus reaction. Within 6–8 hours after inhalation of dust-borne fungal spores, antigen reacts with the IgG present in the lung, initiating an inflammatory reaction which brings in even greater amounts of complement-fixing IgM and IgG. Roitt also cites a similar mechanism for the Arthus-type pulmonary allergy called pigeon-fancier's disease. The antigen involved appears to be serum protein in dried bird feces present in inhaled dust.

Serum sickness occurs 7–10 days after injection of a foreign protein, usually a horse serum antitoxin. The amount of foreign protein is large enough to serve both as the immunogen and to persist in the tissues long enough to function as the eliciting antigen. The acute symptoms of serum sickness are the result of IgE-mediated injury, while the chronic symptoms reflect immune complex-mediated injury resulting from the many interactions of the various foreign serum proteins with the IgM and IgG antibodies which formed in the 7–10 day interval. In the immune complex-mediated injury of serum sickness, immune complexes deposit in the joints and in the kidney glomeruli.

In rare instances, complexes of virus-antibody, hepatitis B antigen (HBAg)-antibody, and even soluble tumor antigen-antibody have been noted to induce immune complex-mediated injury, particularly in the glomeruli.

Poststreptococcal glomerulonephritis occurs within 10–21 days following nasopharyngeal or skin infections by several members of the group A beta hemolytic streptococci (nephritogenic strains). Even though viable streptococci are not cultivated from patients at the time of the glomerulonephritis, pathologic observations (Fig. 9–5) support the contention that soluble complexes of antigen, antibody and complement pass through the pores of the fenestrated endothelium to the basement membrane. These deposits are retained in a subepithelial position, forming humps. In attempts to reach the deposits polymor-

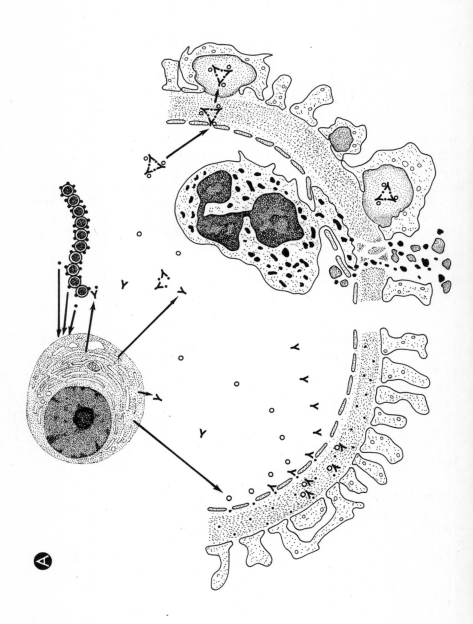

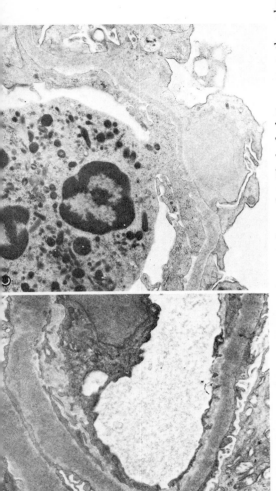

Fig. 9-5.—Mechanism of immune complex-mediated injury. **A**, Schematic representation redrawn from original diagram of R. Fresco. Membrane antigens (●) from a chain of streptococci (*upper right*) stimulate plasma cell (*upper left*) to secrete antistreptococcal immunoglobulin (**Y**) which bind to the antigen and to complement (**O**), forming soluble immune complexes. These circulating complexes reach the glomeruli of the kidney, cross the fenestrated capillary endothelium and basement membrane, and are trapped in the form of subepithelial humps (*right*). The complexes are chemotactic and attract polymorphonuclear leukocytes (both neutrophils and eosinophils). In their attempt to phagocytize the complexes, the leukocytes send pseudopods through the endothelial fenestrae and lift the endothelium from the basement membrane (**C**). Unable to cross the membrane, they discharge their lysosomal granules. The hydrolytic enzymes thus released attempt to break down the complexes, and in the process digest portions of the basement membrane (**A**, *right*). Rarely, the immune deposits may appear in an even linear distribution within the basement membrane (**B**). Several theories have been advanced to explain this. The linearity may be due to entrapment of a particular size of immune deposits within the basement membrane, or it may be due to the formation of antibodies directed against the basement membrane itself. This could be the result of digested fragments of basement membrane being released into the circulation and acting as antigen, or to antigenic cross-reactivity between membrane antigens of certain strains of streptococcus and the glomerular basement membrane (**A**, *left*).

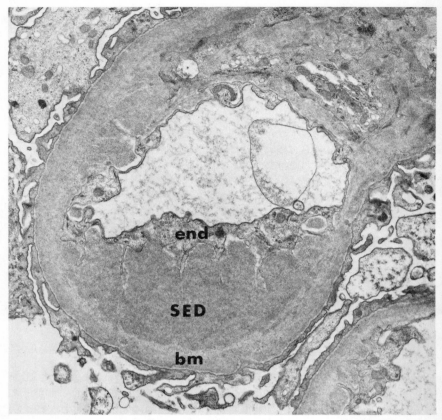

Fig. 9-6.—Immunologically mediated glomerular injury in systemic lupus erythematosus (SLE). In SLE the immune complexes of DNA, anti-DNA and complement accumulate predominantly between the basement membrane (*bm*) of the glomerulus and the endothelium (*end*), in the form of subendothelial deposits (*SED*).

phonuclear neutrophils extrude pseudopods and release lysosomal enzymes which digest away small areas of the basement membrane allowing the passage of blood cells and proteins into the urine. Usually, this disease is acute and self-limiting. When antigen is no longer available, complexes are not generated. If the renal damage were due to antibody reactive both with glomerular basement membrane and nephritogenic streptococci, i.e., antibody reactive with heterogenetic antigens, the immunofluorescent tissue reaction of the kidney glomeruli should show linear deposition of immunoglobulin and complement. In reality, only little of the linear deposits are visible in kidney biopsy specimens from children with acute poststreptococcal glomerulonephritis. In contrast, Goodpasture's syndrome, the etiology of which is unknown, is characterized by the linear deposition of IgG and C3 on the glomerular basement membrane and along the basement membrane of the pulmonary alveolar septae and capillaries. The specificity of IgG eluted from the kidneys is directed against basement membrane antigens of the glomeruli. Antibodies eluted from either the kidneys or lungs will bind to the basement membranes of either the glomeruli or pulmonary alveolar septae.

The kidney damage, central nervous system involvement and skin rash of systemic lupus erythematosus (SLE) are the result of the formation of immune complexes of DNA, anti-DNA and complement. The subsequent injury is again performed by the polymorphonuclear neutrophils. Since the DNA antigen is a large molecular substance, immune complexes of DNA and antibody (IgM and/or IgG) are usually retained in a subendothelial position but may eventually cross the basement membrane and form humps. The lysosomal enzymes released by phagocytes assault the integrity of the basement membrane. These events are shown in Figure 9–6.

Antigens localized in the mesangium are able to react with circulating antibody. Serum IgA can bind to these antigens; aggregated immunoglobulins of any H-chain class can activate the properdin system. Deposits of IgA, properdin and C3 have been described by Peters in association with IgG, on occasion, in glomerular mesangium of patients with focal proliferative glomerulonephritis and recurrent hematuria and in patients with Henoch-Schönlein syndrome.

TYPE IV—CELL MEDIATED
(DELAYED TYPE HYPERSENSITIVITY) INJURY

At this time, the significance of cell-mediated immune (CMI) injury is being actively explored. The three prototypes of cell-mediated immune injury are: initiation of allograft rejection, graft-versus-host reaction and delayed hypersensitivity. As discussed previously, the specifically sensitized T lymphocyte interacts with antigen and the lymphokine effector molecules are released (Figs. 9–7 and 9–8). In CMI injury, the lymphotoxin is the most likely effector molecule to induce necrosis of target cells; other CMI injuries appear to result from a direct interaction of the membranes of the T cell with the specific antigens of the target cell. Cytochalasin B inhibits the adsorption of lymphocytes to target cells. Since cytochalasin B has been shown to

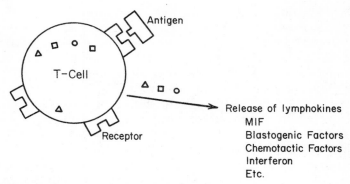

Fig. 9-7.—Mechanism of antigen-mediated release of chemical mediators (lymphokines) from a T lymphocyte in cell-mediated immune injury (delayed type hypersensitivity).

inhibit microfilament formation and subsequent pseudopod formation and cell motion, Henney and Bubbers suggest that membrane modulation of the T cell to expose the antigen recognition site is necessary for the fitting of antigen to the T cell receptor site. If so, the difficulty in identifying the nature of the T cell antigen receptor is better appreciated. However, active metabolic processes are necessary for lymphocyte-mediated cytolysis of target cells. Prostaglandin E and colchicine

Fig. 9-8.—Delayed type hypersensitivity. Footpad response 48 hours after antigen injection in immunized mouse. An extensive mononuclear cell infiltrate is present in the dermis.

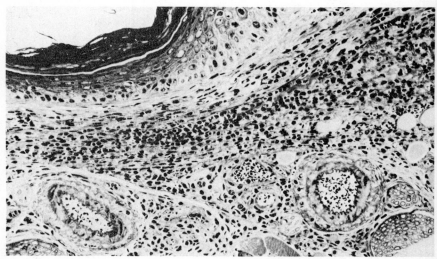

inhibit this cytolysis but do not block adsorption of lymphocytes to target cells.

Most contact dermatitis is T cell-mediated. Many substances, from metals such as nickel to complex chemicals, are capable of inducing contact dermatitis. Since involvement of the established mechanisms of immunologic injury is unclear in many so-called autoimmune disorders such as rheumatic fever (one of the poststreptococcal sequelae), the role of CMI injury needs to be examined. For example, even though IgM, IgG, IgA and complement components have been observed by immunofluorescent staining of cardiac tissue from autopsy specimens of children with rheumatic fever, the immune complex mechanism of injury remains unproved. In general, rheumatic fever patients show normal or elevated serum complement levels, a fact which argues against the mechanism of immune complex disease. The Aschoff nodule, a pathologic hallmark of rheumatic fever, never contains immunofluorescent globulins or complement. Is the Aschoff nodule the remnant of a CMI injury? Roitt advocates that all organ-specific autoimmune injury may be initiated by T cells much as allograft rejection is initiated. Galindo and colleagues have shown that fusion of normal rabbit alveolar macrophages can be induced by a lymphokine (fusion factor) elaborated by BCG-sensitized lymph node cells and antigen.

ANTIBODY-MEDIATED STIMULATION AS A MECHANISM OF IMMUNE INJURY

Presently, only one example exists in which antibody stimulates target cells to overproduce a normal product (type V injury). This

Fig. 9-9.—Proposed mechanisms of antibody-mediated stimulatory injury. Long-acting thyroid stimulator (*LATS*) binds to or near thyroid-stimulating hormone (*TSH*) receptors on thyroid cell causing constant production of T_4 hormone (L-thyroxine).

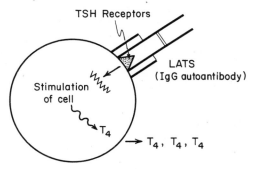

antibody is an IgG immunoglobulin which is synonymous with long-acting thyroid stimulator (LATS). LATS exerts an action on the membrane of thyroid cells similar to that of thyroid-stimulating hormone (TSH), stimulating T_4 hormone production by thyroid cells as diagrammed in Figure 9–9. In contrast to TSH, LATS is not under the control of the pituitary-thyroid axis and patients with LATS exhibit thyrotoxicosis (Graves' disease).

SUGGESTED READINGS

Becker, E. L.: Nature and classification of immediate-type allergic reactions, Adv. Immunol. 13:267, 1971.

Bennett, J. C.: The role and character of immunoglobulins in rheumatoid inflammation, Fed. Proc. 32:138, 1973.

Cochrane, C. G., and Koffler, D.: Immune complex disease in experimental animals and man, Adv. Immunol. 16:186, 1973.

Galindo, B., Lazdins, J., and Castillo, R.: Fusion of normal rabbit alveolar macrophages induced by supernatant fluids from BCG-sensitized lymph node cells after elicitation by antigen, Infect. Immunol. 9:212, 1974.

Gell, P. G. H., and Coombs, R. R. A.: *Clinical Aspects of Immunology,* Section IV (Oxford: Blackwell Scientific Publications, 1968).

Henney, C. S., and Bubbers, J. E.: Antigen-T lymphocyte interactions: inhibition by cytochalasin B, J. Immunol. 111:85, 1973.

Johansson, S. G. O., Bennich, H. H., and Berg, T.: The clinical significance of IgE, Prog. Clin. Immunol. 1:157, 1972.

Lawrence, H. S.: Mediators of cellular immunity, Transplant. Proc. V:49, 1973.

Leddy, J. P., and Swisher, S. N.: Acquired Immune Hemolytic Disorders, in Samter, M. (ed.): *Immunological Diseases,* Vol. II (2nd ed.; Boston: Little, Brown and Company, 1971), p. 1083.

Levis, W. R., Whalen, J. J., and Miller, A. E., Jr.: Blastogenesis of autologous, allogeneic, and syngeneic (identical twins) lymphocytes in response to lymphokines generated in dinitrochlorobenzene-sensitive human leucocyte cultures, J. Immunol. 112:1488, 1974.

Oldstone, M. B. A., and Dixon, F. J.: Mechanisms of Virus-Induced Immunopathology, in Amos, B. (ed.): *Progress in Immunology I* (New York: Academic Press, 1971), p. 763.

Orange, R. P., and Austen, K. F.: The Immunological Release of Chemical Mediators of Immediate Type Hypersensitivity from Human Lung, in Amos, B. (ed.): *Progress in Immunology I* (New York: Academic Press, 1971), p. 173.

Peters, D. K.: The immunologic basis of glomerulonephritis, Proc. Roy. Soc. Med. 67:557, 1974.

Roitt, I. M.: *Essential Immunology* (Oxford: Blackwell Scientific Publications, 1971).

Rothfield, N., *et al.*: Glomerular and dermal deposition of properdin in systemic lupus erythematosus, N. Engl. J. Med. 287:681, 1972.

Roy, L. P., *et al.*: Etiologic agents of immune-deposit disease, Prog. Clin. Immunol. 1:1, 1972.

Ruddy, S., and Austen, K. F.: Activation of the complement system in rheumatoid synovitis, Fed. Proc. 32:134, 1973.

Samter, M. (ed.): *Immunological Diseases*, Vols. I and II (2nd ed.; Boston: Little, Brown and Company, 1971).

Schwartz, R. S.: Therapeutic strategy in clinical immunology, N. Engl. J. Med. 280:367, 1969.

Turk, J. L.: *Immunology in Clinical Medicine* (New York: Appleton-Century-Crofts, 1969).

Ziff, M.: Pathophysiology of rheumatoid arthritis, Fed. Proc. 32:131, 1973.

Zvaifler, N. J.: The immunopathology of joint inflammation in rheumatoid arthritis, Adv. Immunol. 16:265, 1973.

10 / Autoimmunity

Autoimmunization involves the recognition of self antigens by the immune system and may be considered as the loss of immunologic tolerance to self antigens. Immune reactants (antibody and/or cell-mediated immunity) against self antigens may result from (1) the alteration of self antigens, (2) a deficient immune system, or (3) both. The mere presence in an individual of antibody directed against self antigens, i.e., autoantibody, does not necessarily imply concomitant existence of autoimmune disease in that individual. An autoimmune disease is a condition in which structural or functional damage is produced by the reaction of immune cells and/or antibodies with normal body components.

Autoimmune diseases occur more frequently in women (but do occur in men) and in adults more frequently than in children. An increased incidence of both autoimmune and malignant diseases coincides with normal aging and in those individuals born with immunodeficiency diseases. In an evaluation of the antigenic reactivity present in 55 red cell eluates from patients with acquired hemolytic anemia of the warm type, Vos and colleagues found antibodies directed against well-defined Rh system antigens as well as against partially and fully deleted Rh red cell antigens. These observations suggest that the autoimmune disease followed the immune recognition of the modified structural components coded for by the Rh genome in individuals with apparently normally functioning immune systems. Autoantibodies directed against a variety of self antigens are more readily detected in the sera of healthy older individuals. Consequently, it seems that autoimmune diseases may result from either the alteration of self antigens or deficits in the immunologic apparatus.

A classification of the major autoimmune diseases is presented in Table 10–1. The antigenic specificities of the autoantibodies found in each are listed. A partial listing of organ-specific autoimmune diseases is included, as are examples of autoimmune states in which altered self antigens have been identified.

Roitt classifies the autoimmune diseases along a spectrum. At one

TABLE 10-1.—Classification of Autoimmune Diseases

A. Generalized—Accessible Self Antigens
   1. Rheumatoid arthritis
      a. Rheumatoid factor—IgM antibody reactive
         with denatured IgG molecules
   2. Acquired autoimmune hemolytic anemia
      a. Erythrocyte antigens—some are Rh system
         antigens (defect may be in expression of Rh
         genes = "altered self")
   3. Systemic lupus erythematosus (SLE)
      a. Nucleic acid antigens
         (1) DNA
         (2) DNA protein
         (3) Histone
         (4) RNA (double-stranded RNA which is not typical
             of single-stranded mammalian RNA's but is
             characteristic of replicating viral RNA's)
   4. Idiopathic thrombocytopenia purpura—platelets
B. Organ-Specific
   1. Hashimoto's thyroiditis—thyroglobulin, thyroid
      colloid, microsomes, cell surface
   2. Thyrotoxicosis (Graves' disease)—cell surface
   3. Allergic encephalitis—brain and CNS
   4. Allergic neuritis—peripheral nerve
   5. Allergic orchitis and aspermatogenesis—sperm,
      seminal fluid
   6. Uveitis—lens, uvea
   7. Myasthenia gravis—skeletal and heart muscle,
      nuclear and thyroid antigens, thymus myoepithelial
      cells
   8. Pernicious anemia
      a. Intrinsic factor
      b. Parietal cell organelles (microsomes)
   9. Addison's disease—adrenal cell cytoplasm
C. Altered Self Antigens
   1. Heterogenetic antigens—infectious agents containing
      antigens similar or identical to those of humans
      a. Poststreptococcal sequelae
         (1) Rheumatic fever
         (2) Glomerulonephritis
      b. Gram-negative enterics (E. coli)
         (1) Ulcerative colitis
   2. Drug-induced (drug-red cell, drug-platelet, drug-
      white cell, and drug-protein complexes)
      a. Certain purpuras, e.g., thrombocytopenia purpura
      b. Penicillin—induced hemolytic anemias

extreme are the organ-specific autoimmune diseases in which the
lesion involves a specific organ and antibodies to antigen characteristic
of that organ are present in the patient. In addition to the organ-
specific autoimmune diseases listed in Table 10–1, Roitt places the few
cases of premature menopause and certain cases of male infertility in

this category. In the center of the spectrum are diseases in which lesions are localized to one organ but accompanying autoantibodies are not organ-specific. Examples of this mid-spectrum type of autoimmune disease are Goodpasture's disease (see Chapter 9), autoimmune atrophic gastritis, primary biliary cirrhosis (in which the primary site of injury is the small bile ductule, yet autoantibodies are directed against mitochondria), pemphigoid (antibodies to basement membrane), and pemphigus vulgaris (antibodies to desmosomes between prickle cells in epidermis). At the other end of the spectrum are the non-organ-specific autoimmune diseases consisting of systemic lupus erythematosus (SLE), dermatomyositis, scleroderma and rheumatoid arthritis.

Other so-called autoimmune diseases and syndromes exist in the human species. The overlap in classification reflects the tendency for more than one autoimmune disease to exist in the same individual. Even though autoimmune diseases appear in some families, controversy exists as to whether susceptibility to these diseases is a heritable characteristic. Roitt considers hemolytic anemia as a mid-spectrum disease along with ulcerative colitis and Sjögren's syndrome (consisting of symptoms of SLE, rheumatoid arthritis, thyroiditis and dry mucosal surfaces). Patients with Sjögren's syndrome often lack sufficient tears, and gastric (atrophic gastritis) and salivary secretions. Antibodies directed against ducts, mitochondria, nuclei, thyroid and altered IgG have been identified in Sjögren's patients. Granulomatous colitis (Crohn's disease) is a clinical entity, distinct but sometimes difficult to distinguish clinically from ulcerative colitis.

POSSIBLE ETIOLOGIC MECHANISMS OF AUTOIMMUNE DISEASE

For years, the likelihood that the body could mount an immunologic attack against self antigens was held untenable. Erlich had advanced the concept of "horror autotoxicus" which advocated that the immune response was mobilized to react only against foreign antigens and not against self-components; i.e., the body was immunologically incapable of self-destruction. Yet autoimmune diseases do exist in which afflicted individuals manifest not only immunologic reactivity (antibody and/or sensitized T cells) against self antigens but also evidence of immunologic injury.

On a theoretical level, it has been argued that the loss of certain T cell functions, namely, suppressor activity for antigen recognition, occurs as a function of aging. Bretscher has offered a model for the induction of generalized autoimmunity based on the hypothesis that the induction of antibody synthesis requires the interaction of two cells (B and T cells), each bearing receptors which recognize antigen; immune tolerance occurs when antigen binds to the receptors on a single cell. Two signals on the membrane of the B cell are required for the induction of antibody formation whereas one such signal induces tolerance. Bretscher refers to the requirement for the recognition of two determinants on an antigen for the induction of antibody as the principle of "associative recognition." In generalized autoimmunity he predicts that antibodies to thymus antigens are induced prior to the induction of other autoantibodies. As the disease progresses, autoimmune T cell responses also develop against B cell antigens. As a consequence, such T cells would be able to convert a tolerogenic signal by a foreign antigen into an inductive signal for the B cells. The signal would be the second signal for the specific B cells to which tolerogen is bound (signal 1). The B cells subsequently differentiate and antibody is produced. The most likely agent effecting the alteration of thymus antigenicity is a virus. The existence of autoantibodies in patients with immunodeficiency diseases has been postulated to result from the lack of a suppressor T cell population.

MICROBIAL AGENTS AS INDUCERS OF AUTOIMMUNITY

Since certain viruses are immunosuppressive and others remain for long periods of time within host cells (oncogenic viruses and slow viruses), viral agents are currently considered to be the most likely inducers of autoimmune disease. They appear to have the potential to alter both the host immunologic apparatus as well as to modify self antigens. (A modified self-component may be referred to as a "self + X" alteration.)

Virus-induced immunopathology may result from (1) an infection of the immune system with subsequent alteration of immune function, (2) formation of circulating complexes of virus and antibody leading to complement-activated immune complex disease and inflammatory injury, (3) interaction of antibody and complement with virus-induced cell surface antigens, leading to cytotoxic destruction of the infected cells and (4) interaction of immune cells (sensitized T cells and macrophages) with the infected and altered host cells with subsequent release of lymphokines and cytotoxic destruction. The latter two processes may be considered as autoimmune events since the host injury may be mediated by either antibody or T cells directed against "self + X" antigenic configurations.

SLOW VIRUSES AND AUTOIMMUNITY

Certain viral agents are associated with chronic persistent disease. Such host-parasite relationships seem to occur in several progressive central nervous system (CNS) diseases including Creutzfeldt-Jakob disease, kuru, subacute sclerosing panencephalitis (SSPE) and progressive multifocal leukoencephalopathy. The so-called slow virus infections exhibit a prolonged initial period of incubation with a protracted course after the appearance of clinical signs. The usual outcome of these infections is a serious disease and eventual death of the patient. The pathology of the brain of kuru patients is similar to that seen in sheep with scrapie, also a degenerative disease of the CNS. The scrapie agent has been isolated and is filterable; both the kuru agent and that responsible for Creutzfeldt-Jakob disease seem to be filterable, transmissible and extremely small in size. Kuru was present only in the Fore people of New Guinea, especially in females who participated in ceremonial ritual cannibalism; the incidence of kuru has declined precipitously since the cannibalistic rituals have ceased. Although rare, Creutzfeldt-Jacob disease occurs throughout the world. Gajdusek and Gibbs have designated kuru, Creutzfeldt-Jakob disease, scrapie and transmissible mink encephalopathy (TME) as subacute spongiform encephalopathies, since lesions are located principally in the gray matter with vacuole formation in neurons and with the proliferation of certain glial cells; the cerebral cortex acquires a spongy appearance.

The agents of these human and animal diseases are unusual types of "viruses" in that they are resistant to inactivation by ultraviolet irradiation, formalin or heat, but are rendered noninfective by ether or phenol. As yet, they have not been viewed by electronmicroscopy and are thus considered to be extremely small. Certain investigators have speculated that these unconventional agents may be similar to plant viroids (self-replicating RNA molecules of low molecular weight, 50,000). Gajdusek suggests that certain CNS changes attributed to normal aging may actually be the result of virus-induced cell injury.

An agent resembling the measles (rubeola) virus or a defective measles virus has been associated with the pathogenesis of SSPE. In contrast to the other unconventional slow viruses, the agent associated with SSPE resembles the measles virus in electron microscopic examinations of the brains of SSPE patients. As a clinical entity, SSPE develops in individuals from 4 to 20 years of age long after an uncomplicated case of measles. Fields has listed three features of clinical SSPE which implicate the measles virus as a possible etiologic agent: the presence of high titers of antibody to measles virus in spinal fluid; the presence of paramyxovirus-like tubular structures within brain cells of afflicted patients; and the inability to isolate an infectious agent directly from the brains of these patients. He also notes that similar tubular inclusions have been observed in renal biopsies of SLE patients and in patients with other autoimmune diseases. The measles virus may be altered by an abnormal immune response on the part of the host, or more likely, the agent inducing SSPE may actually be a variant or a mutant of the measles virus. Fields believes that double-coated viruses such as measles or herpes virus are agents which may persist in this manner since they would be capable of mutation. In conjunction with this concept is the fact that SSPE has even developed in children who had previously been exposed only to measles vaccine.

Agents such as the slow viruses or the measles-like SSPE agent may well alter host cell antigens in their chronic persistence within host cells. Delayed-type hypersensitive skin responses as well as macrophage migration inhibition and lymphocytes reactive with measles virus have been described in SSPE patients. Mizutani points out that SSPE patients exhibit a higher negative skin test response to measles virus than do persons who have had measles and have not developed SSPE. Other investigators have described the occurrence of aggressive lymphocytes specific for measles in SSPE patients. Consequently, Mizutani suggests that SSPE develops with a gradual emergence of aggressive lymphocytes (cell-mediated immunity) as immunologic tolerance to the measles virus is broken. The immunologic response of SSPE patients to measles virus as well as the role of the T cell in the pathogenesis of SSPE are as yet unresolved.

For many years, speculation has occurred concerning the temporal association of an antecedent virus infection with the development of autoimmune diseases including diabetes mellitus. The virus most often implicated in the genesis of diabetes mellitus in humans has been mumps virus and more recently coxsackie B4 virus. Encephalomyocarditis virus is capable of inducing a diabetic condition in mice. Boucher and Notkins suggest that a virus which even subtly damages the pancreas would be likely to induce the complex virus-host interactions leading to diabetes mellitus.

The involvement of cell-mediated immune reactions (delayed hypersensitivity) in the pathology of organ-specific autoimmune diseases such as myasthenia gravis is suggested by the observations that small lymphocytes are seen in close proximity to necrotic muscle fibers in specimens examined from myasthenic patients. Also, small lymphocytes are associated with the dystrophic abnormality seen in the terminal twigs of peripheral nerves. By immunofluorescent staining procedures, these patients were found to have serum antibodies which bind to the muscle fibers in sections of animal muscle; the lack of detectable antibody at the myoneural junctions of the patients is difficult to explain. In the genesis of organ-specific autoimmune diseases such as myasthenia gravis, the presence of serum autoantibodies may reflect the induction of B cell responses to self antigens following the breaking of T cell tolerance to that antigen. For example, viral alteration of membrane antigens on thymic myoepithelial cells might yield a "self + X" antigenic alteration. Consequently, the T cells recognize the altered self antigen and may then actually collaborate with the B cell system in the induction of antibody to the modified self antigen. Such a series of events may well precede the existence of serum autoantibodies reactive with muscle, thyroid and nuclear antigens in myasthenia gravis patients. Similarly, recent evidence has accumulated to implicate immune T cells reactive with thyroid antigen in the pathogenesis of both Hashimoto's thyroiditis and Graves' disease.

Certain bacteria of the Bedsonia and Mycoplasma species have been implicated as etiologic agents of autoimmune diseases; e.g., Reiter's syndrome. This syndrome, occurring usually in young males, is a clinical triad consisting of urethritis, conjunctivitis and arthritis with occasional mucocutaneous abnormalities. Bedsonia, mycoplasma and viruses have all been associated with this disease, but no convincing evidence establishing a microbial etiology yet exists. Both Mycoplasma species and Bedsonia species have been isolated from synovial and urethral specimens of afflicted patients, but certain of these same bacteria have also been cultured from specimens of apparently healthy individuals. Some patients exhibit elevated titers of serum antibodies to myxoviruses and over half of the patients with Reiter's syndrome produce antibodies to prostate tissue. However, these antibody specificities are not confined to patients with Reiter's syndrome. Autoimmune phenomena have been associated with a variety of other microbial diseases such as tuberculosis, syphilis, gonorrhea, histoplasmosis, malaria, etc.

Patients with malaria, a protozoan infection, sometimes develop autoantibodies directed against self-components such as liver and kidney as well as rheumatoid factor and elevated levels of gamma globulin. Occasionally, immune complex-mediated glomerulonephritis is seen in malaria patients.

Is it merely a reflection of the coincidental distribution of heterogenetic antigens that the cell membranes and walls of most group A beta-hemolytic streptococci share a common antigenicity with the human glomerular basement membrane? Do some individuals inherit the capacity, expressed through T cells, to immunologically recognize these antigens in combination with the myriad of foreign antigens which comprise the bacteria but to remain tolerant to that antigen as it resides on their own tissues?

Since the association between the HL-A histocompatibility type and the tendency to develop poststreptococcal "autoimmune" disease has been observed, it is likely that these individuals may be displaying an unfortunate immune response (ImR) gene function, namely, the capacity to recognize a self-antigen on a foreign carrier cell.

In recent years, support has been gathered for the concept that autoimmune diseases are immunodeficiency diseases. In some cases, a viral etiology has been postulated, infection purportedly initiated by entry via the gut in individuals with secretory IgA deficiency. In support of this contention, many individuals with autoimmune disease have serum antibodies to food proteins (milk and beef). It is argued that the localized secretory IgA system normally functions to protect the host from systemic immunization to antigens (food and microbial) in the gut. When the IgA system is deficient, this barrier is broken as attested to by the existence of serum antibodies directed against dietary proteins. In the same manner, a viral agent could penetrate and, in some way, induce autoimmune disease. However, many people with an apparently intact secretory immunoglobulin system also develop autoimmune disease.

Individuals with deficiencies in complement components appear to be susceptible not only to infectious disease agents but also to the development of autoimmune disease. For example, an increased frequency of infection and an increased incidence of systemic lupus erythematosus, renal diseases, bacterial infections and other connective tissue disorders have been seen in patients with C2 deficiency. C1r deficiency is accompanied by increased susceptibility to infections, renal disease, and dermatitis. Patients with severe combined immunodeficiencies or the X-linked type of agammaglobulinemia also show C1q deficiency; successful bone marrow transplants have restored C1q to normal levels in several patients with combined immunodeficiencies.

The evolution of malignancy and autoimmune disease probably represents a multigenic control of susceptibility to a single specific disease entity. The occurrence of HL-A types has been associated statistically with susceptibility to develop Hodgkin's disease, chronic glomerulonephritis, systemic lupus erythematosus (SLE), acute lymphoblastic leukemia, lymphomas, psoriasis and ankylosing spondylitis*; however, these relationships should be viewed with caution.

An animal model exists for the study of a systemic autoimmune disease which resembles systemic lupus erythematosus of the human. The F_1 hybrids (NZB/NZW) of New Zealand Black (NZB) and New Zealand White (NZW) mice develop an autoimmune disease similar to SLE and often die of immune complex-mediated glomerulonephritis. The NZB parental strain mice develop hemolytic anemia and renal disease as they age. These mouse strains also tend to develop malignant disease upon aging. Talal suggests that these mice are infected with a defective virus which alters their genetic endowment, causing an immunologic imbalance leading to either autoimmunity or malignancy. A progressive loss of suppressor T cell function and theta-positive T cells occurs in these mice prior to and during the initiation of autoimmune manifestations. The immune response of 2-month-old NZB/NZW mice to double-stranded RNA (a synthetic polynucleotide) has been shown to be enhanced by the administration of anti-mouse thymocyte serum and this enhancement effect is lost as the mice age, i.e., at 5–6 months. Antithymocyte antibody has been reported to develop spontaneously in these mice. It has been suggested that the early loss of thymic suppressor T cells may permit B cells to respond to a variety of self-antigens including nucleic acids. (Recall that both stimulatory helper and suppressor roles of T cells on antibody responses have been demonstrated, as described in Chapter 7.) Both the NZB/NZW mouse and certain humans with SLE develop antibodies to DNA and double-stranded RNA. Talal suggests that since double-stranded RNA is absent from mammalian cells, the antibody to it may be in response to the replicating form of single-stranded RNA viruses. A typical virus infection may also be involved in the loss of tolerance to self-antigens in SLE.

The host damage in both SLE and the murine model appears to result from immune complex-mediated injury. Epstein described the immunologic observations in one patient prior to exacerbation of clinical disease. Subsequent attacks of lupus nephritis were preceded by falling levels of serum complement, rising levels of antibody to both single- and double-stranded DNA, and circulating antigen-antibody complexes that bound complement in vitro. These events occurred months prior to clinical evidence of exacerbation of renal

---

*Ankylosing spondylitis is a progressive inflammatory disease of the sacroiliac and synovial joints of the spine with a marked predilection for males. Ninety per cent of patients with ankylosing spondylitis are HL-A W27 positive; this disease has been linked with Reiter's syndrome.

disease. Epstein suggests that abnormal metabolism of immunoglobulin L chains is an early and significant clue to the exacerbation of the nephritis, since this observation reflects the loss of catabolic capabilities of tubule cells. Not all patients with SLE exhibit renal involvement. SLE patients whose predominant antinuclear antibody is directed against the RNA antigen appear not to develop renal complications. As indicated in Table 10–1, an array of antinuclear antibodies has been identified in these patients.

DRUG-INDUCED AUTOIMMUNITY

Drugs, antibiotics in particular, may induce any or several of the four classic types of immunologic injury (see Chapter 9). Many, if not all, drugs bind to serum proteins such as albumin or to particulate elements such as leukocytes, platelets and erythrocytes. This abnormality is detected by the presence of Bence-Jones proteinuria. In all individuals treated with penicillin, the drug is carried throughout the blood stream bound to erythrocytes or to serum proteins. Yet only a small minority of penicillin-treated individuals ever develop penicillin-induced hemolytic anemia or anaphylactic reactions. Why? Is this fact a reflection of a genetic characteristic of the host? For example, do individuals who develop penicillin-induced hemolytic anemia inherit T cells capable of recognizing the combination of "self + drug" and thereby undergo induction of antibody responses by B cells which would be rendered tolerant in the absence of such T cells?

Certain anti-epileptic drugs which exert abnormal alterations of lymphoid tissue are able to exacerbate or initiate episodes of active disease in SLE patients. Unrelated drugs such as sulfa drugs and penicillin may also initiate active disease in an SLE patient whose disease is quiescent.

SUGGESTED READINGS

Alper, C. A., and Rosen, F. S.: Genetic aspects of the complement system, Adv. Immunol. 14:252, 1971.

Amor, B., et al.: HL-A antigen W27—a genetic link between ankylosing spondylitis and Reiter's syndrome? N. Engl. J. Med. 90:572, 1974.

Andres, G., Spiele, H., and McCluskey, R. T.: Viruslike structures in systemic lupus erythematosus, Prog. Clin. Immunol. 1:23, 1972.

Barnes, E. W., and Irvine, W. J.: Clinical syndromes associated with thymic disorders, Proc. Roy. Soc. Med. 66:151, 1973.

Becker, E. L., and Henson, P. M.: In vitro studies of immunologically induced secretion of mediators from cells and related phenomena, Adv. Immunol. 17:94, 1973.

Belohradsky, B. H., *et al.*: Meeting report of the second international workshop on primary immunodeficiency diseases in man, Clin. Immunol. Immunopathol. 2:281, 1974.

Bitter, T., Mottironi, W. D., and Terasaki, P. I.: HL-A antigens associated with lupus erythematosus, N. Engl. J. Med. 286:435, 1972.

Boucher, D. W., and Notkins, A. L.: Virus-induced diabetes mellitus. I. Hyperglycemia and hypoinsulinemia in mice infected with encephalomyocarditis virus, J. Exp. Med. 137:1226, 1973.

van Boxel, J. A.: Multiple heavy-chain determinants on individual B lymphocytes in the peripheral blood of patients with Sjögren's syndrome, N. Engl. J. Med. 289:823, 1973.

Bretscher, P.: A model for generalized autoimmunity, Cell. Immunol. 6:1, 1973.

Bretscher, P. A., and Cohn, M.: A theory of self-nonself discrimination, Science 169:1042, 1970.

Brown, I. N.: Immunological aspects of malaria infection, Adv. Immunol. 11:267, 1969.

Cantor, H., Asofsky, R., and Talal, N.: Synergy among lymphoid cells mediating the graft-vs.-host response. I. Synergy in graft-vs.-host reactions produced by cells from NZB/Bl mice, J. Exp. Med. 131:223, 1970.

Christian, C. L., and Phillips, P. E.: Viruses and autoimmunity, Am. J. Med. 54:611, 1973.

Chused, T. M., Steinberg, A. D., and Parker, L. M.: Enhanced antibody response of mice to polyinosinic-polycytidylic acid by antithymocyte serum and its age-dependent loss in NZB/W mice, J. Immunol. 111:52, 1973.

Cooper, M. D., *et al.*: Meeting report of the second international workshop on primary immunodeficiency diseases in man, Clin. Immunol. Immunopathol. 2:416, 1974.

Dausset, J.: Correlation between histocompatibility antigens and susceptibility to illness, Prog. Clin. Immunol. 1:183, 1972.

Doniach, D.: Autoimmunity in liver diseases, Prog. Clin. Immunol. 1:45, 1972.

Epstein, W. V.: Immunologic events preceding clinical exacerbation of systemic lupus erythematosus, Am. J. Med. 54:631, 1973.

Farid, N. R., *et al.*: Peripheral thymus-dependent (T) lymphocytes in Graves's disease and Hashimoto's thyroiditis, N. Engl. J. Med. 288:1313, 1973.

Finley, S. C., *et al*: Immunological profile in a chromosome 18 delection syndrome with IgA deficiency, J. Med. Gen. 6:388, 1969.

Fudenberg, H. H.: Are Autoimmune Diseases Immunologic Deficiency States? in Good, R. A., and Fisher, D. W. (eds.): *Immunobiology* (Stamford, Conn.: Sinauer Associates, Inc., Publishers, 1971), P. 175.

Glasser, D. L., and Silvers, W. K.: Genetic determinants of immunological responsiveness, Adv. Immunol. 18:1, 1974.

Good, R. A., and Rodey, G. E.: IgA deficiency, antigenic barriers and autoimmunity (editorial), Cell. Immunol. 1:147, 1970.

Harris, J. E., and Sinkovics, J. G.: The Immunology of Malignant Disease (St. Louis: The C. V. Mosby Company, 1970).

Hawkins, D.: Clinical Immunology of the Kidney; Clinical Immunology of the Heart, in Freedman, S. O.: Clinical Immunology (New York: Harper & Row Publishers, 1971), P. 152.

Kallick, C. A., et al.: Systemic lupus erythematosus associated with Haemobartonella-like organisms, Nature New Biol. 236:145, 1972.

Marx, J. L.: Slow viruses: Role in persistent disease, Science 181:1351, 1973.

McDevitt, H. O., and Bodner, W. F.: Histocompatibility antigens, immune responsiveness and susceptibility to disease (editorial), Am. J. Med. 52:1, 1972.

McFarlin, D. E.: Myasthenia Gravis, in Samter, M. (ed.): Immunological Diseases, Vol. II (2nd ed.; Boston: Little, Brown and Company, 1971), P. 1150.

Mizutani, H.: Instability of cellular immunity in patients with subacute sclerosing panencephalitis, N. Engl. J. Med. 287:1098, 1972.

Morris, R., et al.: HL-A W27—a clue to the diagnosis and pathogenesis of Reiter's syndrome, N. Engl. J. Med. 290:554, 1974.

Naff, G. B.: Properdin—its biologic importance, N. Engl. J. Med. 287:716, 1972.

Notkins, A., and Koprowski, H.: How the immune response to a virus can cause disease, Sci. Am. 228:22, 1973.

Oldstone, M. B. A., and Dixon, F. J.: Mechanisms of Virus-Induced Immunopathology, in Amos, B. (ed.): Progress in Immunology I. (New York: Academic Press, 1971), p. 763.

Paterson, P. Y.: Multiple sclerosis: An immunologic reassessment, J. Chronic Dis. 26:119, 1973.

Rachelefsky, G. S., et al.: Increased prevalence of W27 in juvenile rheumatoid arthritis, N. Engl. J. Med. 290:892, 1974.

Roitt, I. M.: Essential Immunology (Oxford: Blackwell Scientific Publications, 1971).

Russell, T. J., Schultes, L. M., and Kuban, D. J.: Histocompatibility (HL-A) antigens associated with psoriasis, N. Engl. J. Med. 287:738, 1972.

Russell, W. O. (chairman): Fifth annual ASCP research symposium viruses and autoimmune disease, Am. J. Clin. Pathol. 56:259, 1971.

Sharp, G. C., Mullen, H., and Kyriakos, M.: Production of augmented experimental autoimmune thyroiditis lesions by combined transfer of antiserum and lymph node cells, J. Immunol. 112:478, 1974.

Sigel, M. M., and Good, R. A. (eds.): Tolerance, Autoimmunity and Aging (Springfield, Ill.: Charles C Thomas, Publisher, 1972).

Stutman, O.: Lymphocyte subpopulations in NZB mice: Deficit of thymus-dependent lymphocytes, J. Immunol. 109:602, 1972.

Thomas, L.: Experimental mycoplasma infections as models of rheumatoid arthritis, Fed. Proc. 32:143, 1973.

Thurman, G. B., *et al.*: Lymphocyte activation in subacute sclerosing panencephalitis virus and cytomegalovirus infections, in vitro stimulation in response to viral-infected cell lines, J. Exp. Med. 138:839, 1973.

Vos, G. H., Petz, L. D., and Fudenberg, H. H.: Specificity and immunoglobulin characteristics of autoantibodies in acquired hemolytic anemia, J. Immunol. 106:1172, 1971.

Weiner, L. P., Johnson, R. T., and Herndon, R. M.: Viral Infections and demyelinating diseases, N. Engl. J. Med. 288:1103, 1973.

White, S. H., *et al.*: Disturbance of HL-A antigen frequency in psoriasis, N. Engl. J. Med. 287:740, 1972.

Zeman, W., and Lennette, E. H. (eds.): *Slow Virus Diseases*, American Association of Pathologists and Bacteriologists, 1973 (Baltimore: The Williams and Wilkins Company, 1974).

11 / Tumor and Allograft Immunity

HOST RESPONSES TO TISSUE ANTIGENS

A variety of specific responses may develop in the immune response to tissue antigens. Several types of humoral antibody responses to tissue antigens may occur as well as specific cell-mediated immunity.

Certain antibody molecules bind complement and may bring about the death of cells containing membrane-situated antigens. When these antigens are tumor cell-specific, they are referred to as tumor-specific transplantation antigens (TSTA's). Other antibody molecules directed against membrane-situated antigens do not bind complement but do bind to the histocompatibility (HL-A), TSTA or other antigens on the surface of the cell. These antibodies are referred to as blocking or enhancing antibodies and in the human appear to be 7S IgG-type globulins. A third functional type of humoral response has been described by the Hellströms. Antibodies which specifically abrogated ("unblocked") the blocking effect were found in the sera of mice whose Moloney virus-induced sarcomas had spontaneously regressed.

A specific cell-mediated immune response may also develop and, if permitted to react with cells containing TSTA, brings about their death. Consequently, an antibody and a cell-mediated immunity to tissue antigens exist which are capable of killing cells bearing these antigens.

Enhancing antibody is a term used to describe the antibody which coats allograft antigens thereby preventing rejection; *blocking antibody* is the term used to describe this same activity in which antibody binds to TSTA's and blocks attack by cytotoxic antibody and reactive T cells. When this type of antibody first reaches the cells containing antigen, the destruction by the complement-mediated cytotoxic antibody or by the so-called "killer" T cells is blocked. The existence of F(ab')$_2$ fragments of IgG which have blocking activity has been described in the sera of cancer patients. These fragments were able to inhibit cell-mediated immune reactions in vitro.

In the immunotherapy of cancer the desired immune responses

would involve the generation of "killer" T lymphocytes as well as the production of cytotoxic antibody, both of which would be directed against TSTA's. Immunologically induced cell destruction by five different soluble mediators whose synthesis and/or release is triggered by antigen activation of sensitized T cells has been suggested. However, no clues exist to determine whether these responses occur in the absence of blocking-type antibodies which protect the tumor cells. Both Sjögren and associates, as well as Smith, have argued that the circulating TSTA's play a key role in the efficacy of the host immune response against malignant tumors. For example, combinations of multivalent TSTA and divalent antibody may exert blocking action by "defusing" specifically reactive T cells in the circulation. Reactive T cells bind to available free antigenic sites in the antigen-antibody complexes. Consequently, the effectiveness of the cell-mediated immune response against the tumor cells is diminished. If the deblocking factor can be precisely defined and mobilized efficiently, some reversal of enhancement or blocking may be effected in vivo. The goals of immunotherapy in human malignancy are the opposite of those in transplantation immunology. In transplantation immunity the sole generation of enhancing-type antibody would prevent the destruction of the allograft by cell-mediated and cytotoxic antibody responses.

Recently, several approaches to the immunotherapy of cancer in humans have yielded encouraging results. Mathe's group, Morton, and others have observed that active immunization with BCG and autologous tumor cells induces a heightened immune response against tumor-associated antigens which was sometimes therapeutic. Currently, the utilization of BCG vaccine in the treatment of malignant disease is controversial. Both beneficial and adverse effects on the progression of malignant disease in cancer patients have been observed after BCG administration.

HOST REACTIONS TO ALLOGRAFTED TISSUES

Hyperacute rejection appears to be a complement-mediated immune complex (Arthus) reaction. Some feel that this reaction is a Shwartzman-Sanarelli reaction. In hyperacute rejection, the host response is immediate and results in failure of the graft. The existence of preformed antibodies which are the result of previous transfusions, pregnancy or ABO incompatibility in the recipient is probably the predisposing factor to this type of tissue rejection. The damage which is seen is characteristic of complement-mediated immune complex tissue destruction, in that fibrin deposition, platelet aggregation, microscopic thrombi and infiltration of polymorphonuclear neu-trophils are seen. The antigen-antibody-complement complexes appear to induce the clotting observed. (Recall that activation of the comple-ment cascade is interrelated to the activation of the kinin and coagula-tion cascade reactions.)

Acute rejection is initiated by a cell-mediated immune (CMI) de-layed hypersensitivity type reaction and may involve immune complex damage. This response occurs in the recipient after the sixth day following transplantation and proceeds rapidly once initiated. (An accelerated allograft rejection response which occurs 5 days after transplantation may be a cell-mediated immune response. Acute rejec-tion responses occurring 10–30 days after transplant are initiated by T cells.) Clinically, the transplanted organ loses function. In the recipi-ent local pain and swelling of the graft are accompanied by fever, malaise, leukocytosis and thrombocytopenia. During rejection blood flow to the graft is greatly impaired. Occasionally, decreases in total serum complement levels occur. The involvement of complement may proceed as follows. Complement-binding antibody may attach to antigens on the cells in the graft, activate complement and effect cytotoxicity; circulating antigens may react with antibody in the circulation, bind complement and lead to immune complex deposition and inflammatory injury. The pathologic description of this type of rejection is characterized by infiltration of large numbers of mononu-clear cells typical of cell-mediated immune reactions. However, poly-morphonuclear neutrophils, typical of the inflammatory reaction trig-gered by immune complexes, may also be evident. Acute rejection may lead to complete rejection of the grafted tissue or may be reversed by administering appropriate immunosuppressive therapy.

Chronic rejection is a slow and progressive loss of function of the transplanted organ. This response occurs in spite of the fact that the patients have been undergoing immunosuppressive treatment for prolonged periods. Such treatment must not be totally immunosup-pressive; otherwise the patients would be unable to fend off over-whelming infection by their own microflora. Immunosuppressive agents are discussed in Chapter 12. Although complement-mediated immunologic injury seems to be the primary mechanism of chronic rejection, cell-mediated immune injury also appears to be involved. Hume cites antibody-mediated injury as the mechanism of primary chronic rejection in renal transplants. He has observed that circulating antibody "irritates the intima of the arterial tree producing endothelial proliferation, narrowing of the arterial lumen and reduction of distal blood flow." Furthermore, he has observed that antibody in the glomerular tuft "attaches to the glomerular basement membrane in antigen-antibody complexes," activating complement. Membranous glomerulonephritis results from the complement-mediated injury. Voisin has offered an explanation for the role of cell-mediated immune reactions in chronic allograft rejection. The vascular permeability in the allograft is increased by the circulating antigen-specific T lymphocytes. The increased vascular permeability resulting from the cell-mediated immune reaction in the graft allows the passage of immune agents (complement-fixing antibody, complement and/or complexes of antigen-antibody-complement) into the target tissues. Voisin's explanation is supported by the fact that specific antigraft antibodies when injected intravenously into allograft recipients (experimental animals) usually *cannot* initiate rejection of a solid graft. In chronic rejection the rejected organ is infiltrated with moderate numbers of mononuclear cells indicative of CMI injury. In rejected kidneys both narrowing of the arterial lumen and evidence of membranous glomerulonephritis are seen. Treatment is usually unsatisfactory and complete rejection occurs.

Graft-versus-host reactions result when immunocompetent cells from an allogeneic individual are placed into an immunologically incompetent individual. In the human these reactions have occurred in immunodeficient children in which immunologic reconstitutions have been attempted. They have also been seen in the treatment of erythroblastosis fetalis in which the fetus was transfused in utero with blood containing lymphocytes. T cells present in the grafted lymphoid cell population respond to alloantigens present on the recipient's cells. Thus, a cell-mediated immune response is made against the host cells. The clinical characteristics of this response are anorexia, diarrhea, loss of hair, rash, leukopenia, anemia, thrombocytopenia and death when the reaction is severe.

POSSIBLE INTERRELATIONSHIPS BETWEEN ONCOGENESIS AND HOST IMMUNE SYSTEMS

Thomas and Good have advocated the hypothesis of immunologic surveillance which proposes that normally any clone of malignant cells arising is rapidly rejected as an allograft unless a defect exists in the immune response that allows the malignant cells to be accepted. In a review of this concept, Laroye suggests that a malignant cell clone arises only if that clone contains an antigenic difference for which the immunologic apparatus is not programmed to react efficiently. The inability of T cells to recognize this antigenic difference constitutes a selective defect in immune surveillance. This selective defect may be effected in any one of the following ways. (1) If an individual lacked immune response (ImR) genes for certain determinants of a given TSTA, then the T cell system would not recognize that particular antigenic grouping and the malignant cells would be accepted as self. (2) The failure of recognition of a TSTA by the immune apparatus may involve a temporary inactivation of T cell function during infection by a virus which exhibits a predilection for lymphoid tissues. (3) Based on the observations that leukemias and lymphomas have developed during the course of certain autoimmune diseases (Sjögren's syndrome, autoimmune hemolytic anemia, etc.) and in immunodeficiency states such as congenital agammaglobulinemia, immune disturbances may activate a latent oncogenic virus.

Support for the third possibility was provided by Armstrong and colleagues. A graft-versus-host reaction activated a murine leukemia virus in strains of mice normally exhibiting low spontaneous incidences of lymphoreticular malignancy. A parallel was drawn between their mouse model and Burkitt's lymphoma, a likely counterpart in humans. Burkitt's lymphoma is associated with a herpes-like DNA virus. In Africa, Burkitt's lymphoma is associated with the Epstein-Barr (EB) virus. In tissue culture EB virus morphologically transforms human embryonic fibroblasts, suggesting its oncogenic potential. Burkitt's lymphoma occurs mainly in children in geographic locales where malaria is endemic. Chronic malaria stimulates lymphoreticular hyperplasia and thereby *may* provide the virus with the "lymphoblastoid" cells that it requires for growth. Schwartz has presented an hypothesis which accounts for the development of lymphomas in patients with autoimmunity and in allograft recipients; in addition, the relationship between malaria and lymphomas was examined. He suggests that one of the main evolutionary pressures generating the immunoregulatory mechanism of mammals is the presence of latent oncogenic viruses in lymphocytes. Several groups of investigators have contended that all normal cells possess the necessary genetic information for the assembly of an RNA tumor virus, an "oncogene," or "virogene." Since such latent oncogenic viruses can be activated by the immune response, Schwartz maintains that some mechanism should exist to prevent the expression of the virogene in lymphocytes. He develops this hypothesis using the following information. (1) Graft-versus-host reactions do, indeed, activate latent oncogenic viruses in mice by some as yet unknown molecular mechanism. (2) All steps leading from the immune recognition of the grafted tissue to the emergence of a recognizable lymphoma are probably under genetic control. (3) According to the doctrine of immune surveillance, mutant cells arise often and are promptly destroyed by immune responses directed against their surface antigens. (4) Auto-immune responses in which lymphocytes reactive with self antigens arise may provide the population of transformed lymphocytes within which activation of the virogene can occur. (5) The association of Burkitt's lymphoma with malaria, the high incidence of double neo-plasms in patients receiving chemotherapy, the development of malig-nant lymphomas in patients with autoimmune disease, and the high incidence (100 times expected rate) of neoplasms in recipients of kidney grafts who are partially immunosuppressed with drugs and antilymphocyte sera lend further support to the contention that immu-nologic derangement precedes malignancy.

Schwartz has proposed that "feedback loops" regulating the im-mune response exist which should be able to prevent activation of the "virogene" and its replication in lymphocytes. Therefore, feedback mechanisms which regulate the various aspects of the immune re-sponse are of considerable significance. Defects in the regulation of T cell or B cell responses may lead to lymphoid hyperplasia. For example, in individuals in which immunization is combined with immunosuppressive therapy, selective impairment of the synthesis of IgG antibodies occurs. Thus, immunoregulation is inefficient and lymphoid hyperplasia is sustained.

Additional support for Schwartz' hypothesis has been gathered by Hirsch and associates who observed that murine leukemia viruses were activated in immunosuppressed mice which had received skin allografts. Virus was found in most of the mice that had received both skin allografts and antilymphocyte serum which selectively depresses circulating T cell functions. Virus was not found in mice that had received only antilymphocyte serum alone or only skin allografts; virus was not detected in normal (untreated) mice.

Kalter and associates found C type viral structures in normal baboon placentas at various periods during pregnancy and these structures were curiously prevalent in trophoblasts. Since oncogenic C type virus structures are associated with a variety of tumors and leukemias in animal hosts, these investigators suggest that their observations may support the concept that the protovirus (virogene or cancer-inducing gene) is vertically transmitted.

THE FETUS AS AN ALLOGRAFT?

Even though antibodies directed against paternally endowed char-acteristics may be detected to fetal antigens in multiparous women and female mice, fetuses are not immunologically rejected as allografts.

The physiologic barrier between mother and fetus which prevents allograft rejection is attributed to the nonantigenicity of fetal trophoblasts. The lack of immunogenicity of the fetal trophoblasts within the mother may well be the result of the secretion of fibrinoid by these cells creating an immunologic barrier of the placenta.

HL-A ANTIGENS AND MIXED LEUKOCYTE CULTURE (MLC) ANTIGENS USED IN TISSUE TYPING

The HL-A antigens are one of the major antigen systems against which human immune responses to allografts are directed. The mixed leukocyte culture (locus) is thought to be distinct and different from that of the HL-A alleles. Bach and colleagues consider the major histocompatibility complex (MHC) in man and mouse to consist of two histocompatibility loci; one locus controls the serologically defined antigens of the HL-A system in man and the H-2 system in mice, while the other locus controls the lymphocyte defined (LD) antigens. The cell-mediated T cell responses of the allograft recipient causing donor cell destruction, i.e., the so-called "killer lymphocyte" response, apparently is directed against the HL-A antigens in man and the H-2 antigens in mice.

This "killer lymphocyte" response can be measured in vitro using lymphocytes of both donor and recipient mice. The donor target lymphocytes are first labelled alone with Cr^{51} and then placed in culture with recipient lymphocytes. If the recipient lymphocytes exert cytotoxicity, Cr^{51} is released from the target donor lymphocytes after membrane damage induced by the recipient's "killer lymphocytes." This test cannot be done routinely or practically with human donor and recipient lymphoid cells.

LD antigens are becoming increasingly important in the matching of tissue types. They are measured in the MLC test which is also performed as a mixed lymphocyte culture.

In this test the donor lymphocytes are first treated with mitomycin C to arrest DNA synthesis and cell division; such treated cells are used as test antigen. Treated donor cells are added to untreated recipient lymphocytes in cell culture. After several days in culture, H^3-thymidine is added; the uptake of H^3-thymidine by the recipient cells is usually determined 24 hours later. If LD antigens of the two lymphoid cell populations are alike (identical), no increased uptake of H^3-thymidine is noted; if the LD antigens of the donor and recipient differ, then considerable uptake of H^3-thymidine is seen since the recipient cells are stimulated by the different antigens present on the donor cells used in the test.

HL-A antigens are present on lymphoid cells after long-term culturing. Such cells exhibit a higher density of HL-A determinants than do autologous peripheral blood lymphocytes. Cultured cells also have greater concentrations of "lymphoblast in vitro antigens."

Qualitative and quantitative changes in HL-A antigens may be found after in vitro manipulations such as exposure to chemicals, viral carcinogens or hormones. The emergence of new HL-A antigens has been described during acute phase leukemia. These antigens disappear during remission and reoccur in relapse. In addition to the HL-A and LD antigen systems and the major blood group antigens, other histocompatibility antigen systems probably exist in the human species.

β₂ MICROGLOBULIN, HL-A SYSTEM AND LYMPHOCYTE RECEPTORS

β_2 microglobulin, a small polypeptide (molecular weight of 11,700 daltons), is a membrane-bound protein of human lymphocytes. It appears to be a portion of the HL-A antigen system and is bound to another polypeptide (molecular weight of 45,000) on cell membranes. Purified HL-A antigens contain 20–25% β_2 microglobulin. Thus, the small subunits of the HL-A antigen system seem to be identical to β_2 microglobulin. Also, β_2 microglobulin has been found to share a high degree of homology with certain regions of immunoglobulin molecules. Anti-β_2 microglobulin serum blocks lymphocyte reactivity against allogeneic cells in mixed lymphocyte culture and against stimulation by phytohemagglutinin. Thus, β_2 microglobulin, HL-A antigens and T cell antigen receptors appear to be intimately related. In rats, antireceptor antibody was able to inhibit both T and B cell responses to antigens.

SUGGESTED READINGS

Armstrong, M. Y. K., et al.: Tumor induction by immunologically activated murine leukemia virus, J. Exp. Med. 137:1163, 1973.

Bach, F. H., et al.: Cell-mediated immunity: separation of cells involved in recognition and destructive phases, Science 180:403, 1973.

Bach, M. L., Huang, S.-W., and Hong, R.: β₂-microglobulin: Association with lymphocyte receptors, Science 182:1350, 1973.

Bansal, S. C., and Sjögren, H. O.: "Unblocking" serum activity in vitro in the polyoma system may correlate with antitumour effects of antiserum in vivo, Nature New Biol. 233:76, 1971.

Bansal, S. C., and Sjögren, H. O.: Correlation between changes in antitumor immune parameters and tumor growth in vivo in rats, Fed. Proc. 32:165, 1973.

Billingham, R., and Silvers, W.: The Immunology of Transplantation, Foundations of Immunology Series (Englewood Cliffs, N. J.: Prentice-Hall, Inc., 1971).

Bluming, A. Z.: BCG: A note of caution, N. Engl. J. Med. 289:860, 1973.

TUMOR AND ALLOGRAFT IMMUNITY 195

Cerottini, J.-C., and Brunner, K. T.: Cell-mediated cytotoxicity, allograft rejection and tumor immunity, Adv. Immunol. 18:67, 1974.

Ferrone, S., and Pellegrino, M. A.: HL-A antigens, antibody and complement in the lymphocytotoxic reaction, Contemp. Top. Mol. Immunol. 2:185, 1973.

Fu, S. M., Winchester, R. J., and Kunkel, H. G.: Occurrence of surface IgM, IgD and free light chains in human lymphocytes, J. Exp. Med. 139:451, 1974.

Gold, P.: Human Cancer Immunology; Organ Transplantation, in Freeman, S. O., Clinical Immunology (New York: Harper & Row, 1971), p. 399.

Good, R. A.: Disorders of the Immune System, in Good, R. A., and Fisher, D. W. (eds.): Immunobiology (Stamford, Conn.: Sinauer Associates, Inc., 1971), p. 3.

Grey, H. M., et al.: The small subunit of HL-A antigens in β₂-microglobulin, J. Exp. Med. 138:1608, 1973.

Harris, J. E., and Sinkovics, J. G.: The Immunology of Malignant Disease (St. Louis: The C. V. Mosby Company, 1970).

Hellström, I., and Hellström, K. E.: Some recent studies on cellular immunity to human melanomas, Fed. Proc. 32:156, 1973.

Hellström, K. E., and Hellström, I.: Lymphocyte-mediated cytotoxicity and blocking serum activity to tumor antigens, Adv. Immunol. 18:209, 1974.

Herberman, R. B.: In vivo and in vitro assays of cellular immunity to human tumor antigens, Fed. Proc. 32:160, 1973.

Hirsch, M., et al.: Leukemia virus activation during homograft rejection, Science 180:500, 1973.

Hume, D. M.: Organ Transplants and Immunity, in Good, R. A., and Fisher, D. W. (eds.): Immunobiology (Stamford, Conn.: Sinauer Associates, Inc., 1971).

Kalter, S. S., et al.: Observations of apparent C-type particles in baboon (Papiocynocephalus) placentas, Science 179:1332, 1973.

Kirby, D. R. S.: Transplantation and Pregnancy, in Rapaport, F. T., and Dausset, J. (eds.): Human Transplantation (New York: Grune and Stratton, 1968), p. 565.

Laroye, G. J.: Cancer caused by an inherited selective defect in immunological surveillance, Lancet 1:641, 1973.

Levy, N. L., Mahaley, M. S., Jr., and Day, E. D.: Serum-mediated anti-tumor immunity in a melanoma patient: association with BCG immunotherapy and clinical deterioration, Int. J. Cancer 10:244, 1972.

Mathé, G.: The immunological approach to cancer treatment, J. R. Coll. Physicians Lond. 5:62, 1970.

McKearn, T. J.: Antireceptor antiserum causes specific inhibition of reactivity to rat histocompatibility antigens, Science 183:94, 1974.

Morton, D. L., et al.: Recent advances in oncology, Ann. Intern. Med. 77:431, 1972.

Old, L. J., and Boyse, E. A.: *Current Enigmas in Cancer Research,* in The Harvey Lectures, Series 67 (New York: Academic Press, 1973).

Perlmann, P., O'Toole, C., and Unsgaard, B.: Cell-mediated immune mechanisms of tumor cell destruction, Fed. Proc. 32:153, 1973.

Poulik, M. D., *et al*: Aggregation of HL-A antigens at the lymphocyte surface induced by antiserum to β_2-microglobulin, Science 182:1352, 1973.

Reisfeld, R. A., and Kahan, B. D.: Human histocompatibility antigens, Contemp. Top. Immunochem. 1:51, 1972.

Rosenthal, S. R., *et al.*: BCG vaccination and leukemia mortality, JAMA 228:1543, 1972.

Schwartz, R. S.: Immunoregulation, oncogenic viruses and malignant lymphomas, Lancet 2:1266, 1972.

Sjögren, H. O., *et al.*: Suggestive evidence that the "blocking antibodies" of tumor-bearing individuals may be antigen-antibody complexes, Proc. Nat. Acad. Sci. USA 68:1372, 1971.

Smith, R. T.: Possibilities and problems of immunologic intervention in cancer, N. Engl. J. Med. 287:439, 1972.

Snell, G. D.: The H-2 locus of the mouse: observations and speculations concerning its comparative genetics and its polymorphism, Folia Biol. (Praha) 14:335, 1968.

Sparks, F. C.: Complications of BCG immunotherapy in patients with cancer, N. Engl. J. Med. 289:827, 1973.

Stjernswärd, J., *et al.*: Lymphopenia and change in distribution of human B and T lymphocytes in peripheral blood induced by irradiation for mammary carcinoma, Lancet 1:1352, 1972.

Thomas, L.: Discussion, of Medawar, P. B.: Reactions to Homologous Tissue Antigens and Relation to Hypersensitivity, in Lawrence, H. S. (ed.): *Cellular and Humoral Aspects of the Hypersensitive States* (New York: Hoeber, 1959), pp. 529-532.

Voisin, G. A.: Actions and Interactions of Immunoglobulins in Immune Tissue Damage, in Amos, B.: *Progress in Immunology I.* (New York: Academic Press, 1971), p. 193.

Weiser, R. S., Myrvik, Q. N., and Pearsall, N. N.: *Fundamentals of Immunology, for Students of Medicine and Related Sciences* (Philadelphia: Lea and Febiger, 1969).

12 / Manipulations of the Immune Response

VACCINATION

The term *vaccine* (*vacca* = cow) has been derived from the original observations by Jenner that cowpox virus afforded protection in humans against infection by smallpox (variola) virus. The modified or attenuated virus sharing protective antigens with the variola virus is the vaccinia virus which is used as a vaccine in humans against smallpox. In the strictest sense, vaccination is the process whereby a human or animal host is inoculated with an attenuated virus (by either a single injection or series of injections) for the purpose of stimulating actively acquired immunity against the virulent strain of that virus. (Immunity acquired in this manner is referred to as artificial, actively acquired immunity, see Chapter 1.) Until rather recently (1950's to 1960's) vaccinia virus was the only living attenuated virus agent used in humans. Attempts to stimulate effective immune resistance using dead virus vaccines have, for the most part, been unsuccessful.

In recent years, the use of the term vaccine has been corrupted in that any microorganism or microbial product used as immunogen is often referred to as a vaccine. In this discussion the corrupted use of the term vaccine will be employed.

TYPES OF VACCINES CURRENTLY IN USE

Virus Vaccines

Since the advent of modern cell culture technics, many effective living attenuated virus vaccines have been developed and are available for use in humans, e.g., poliovirus types 1, 2 and 3, measles (rubeola) virus, German measles (rubella) virus, mumps virus and yellow fever virus. Initially, the use of the attenuated polio vaccine developed independently by Sabin and Kaprowsky was met with great resistance, on the fear that each type of poliovirus might revert to its virulent form. In spite of the fact that the vaccinia virus had been used for years and

197

never reverted to a virulent form, the opponents of the living polio vaccine argued that no proof existed that vaccinia virus had ever been virulent or was even derived from the smallpox virus. After a period of time, the fears concerning the use of an attenuated polio vaccine dissipated; the three living polio vaccine strains have not reverted or given rise to a virulent strain. Moreover, the attenuated polioviruses appear to exhibit infectivity for the cells of the gastrointestinal tract and not the spinal cord while virulent polio strains are capable of infecting both types of cells. The attenuated poliovirus strains are able to induce secretory antibody (IgA) response at the initial site of infection of the virulent forms and also to stimulate humoral antibody (IgG mainly but also some IgM and serum IgA) following viremia. As discussed in both Chapters 3 and 8, the significance of stimulating immune resistance at the portal of entry of the virus is more fully appreciated now that we realize the importance of the localized secretory antibody system in host resistance to microbial agents. The role of cell-mediated immune T cell responses in the mucous membrane routes of microbial entry is currently being evaluated in many laboratories.

The 17D strain of yellow fever virus was attenuated through repeated passage in chick embryos and is a highly efficient vaccine imparting immunity of long duration in humans. On the other hand, rabies virus which was passaged by Pasteur in rabbit brains is still used as a killed virus vaccine in humans. Pasteur's virulent agent ("street" rabies virus) is passaged through 20 to 25 rabbits to decrease the pathogenicity for humans ("fixed" virus). The "fixed" rabies virus is inactivated by agents such as phenol or formalin (Semple vaccine) and a series of 14 injections is required in the immunization of humans bitten by a rabid animal (dog, bat, squirrel, etc.). Since the incubation period of rabies is as short as 21 days but often longer, therapeutic immunization is used to treat persons bitten by an animal *proved* to be rabid. Since the Semple type vaccine contains nerve tissue, autoimmune complications such as neuritis and myelitis may occur. Consequently, a rabies vaccine of lesser immunogenicity but greater safety has been developed in duck embryos. The duck embryo rabies virus is killed by treatment with beta-propiolactone. The World Health Organization Expert Committee on Rabies has made the following recommendations.

    I. If contact with the rabid animal has been indirect or if there has been only a lick on unabraded skin, no exposure is considered to have occurred and vaccination is not recommended.

    II. If the exposure was mild, i.e., a lick on abraded skin or on mucosal surfaces, or for single bites *not* on the head, neck, face, or arm:

A. If the animal is healthy at the time of exposure, withhold vaccine, but observe the animal for 10 days.

B. If during the 10-day observation period the animal is proved to have rabies or becomes clinically suspicious, start vaccine immediately.

C. If the animal has signs suspicious of rabies at the time of exposure, start vaccine immediately, but stop injections if the animal is normal on the fifth day after exposure.

D. If the animal is rabid, if it escapes or is killed, or if it is unknown, give complete course of vaccine. If the biting animal is wild, also give rabies antiserum.

III. If exposure was severe (multiple bites or single bites on the head, neck, face or arm), the indications for giving vaccine are the same as those for mild exposure. The administration of rabies antiserum is recommended.*

Smallpox has been eradicated in the United States since 1950 and by 1968 13% of the American population remained unvaccinated and yet no smallpox cases were reported. Since at least 7 deaths per year occur from smallpox vaccination reactions, it is suggested that smallpox vaccination procedures no longer be mandatory in the United States. Yet, smallpox exists in other portions of the world and Americans have become global travelers since World War II. When smallpox vaccination is elected, the following immunization procedure is recommended by the U.S. Public Health Service:

(1) Primary vaccination between a child's first and second birthdays or at any age under conditions of foreign travel,

(2) Revaccination on entering school or kindergarten,

(3) Revaccination at 3-year intervals for persons who may be exposed to smallpox through travel to endemic areas or persons who may be exposed to newly imported cases of the disease such as doctors, hospital workers and morticians,

(4) Routine vaccination at regular 10-year intervals.

The most effective vaccinia vaccines are prepared by inoculating scarified areas of the shaved belly of a calf. Subsequently, the confluent vesicles are removed and emulsified for use as vaccine. The greatest problem with such vaccines is sterility.

---

*Farnsworth cites that serum administered concurrently with vaccine seriously interferes with the development of active immunity. If serum is used, supplementary doses of vaccine ten and twenty days after the last dose in the initial series are recommended.

The use of attenuated rubella virus vaccine imparts an antibody response in virtually all who are vaccinated without a decline in antibody titers for over 2 years. Rubella vaccination of young women in their child-bearing years who have no antibody titer for rubella virus is advocated to prevent severe congenital deformities in fetuses of infected mothers.

The influenza virus vaccines in use are formalin-inactivated viruses purified from the allantoic fluid of virus-inoculated chick embryos. About 20% of the individuals receiving this vaccine developed side-effects from the egg proteins. These side-effects have been diminished by a further purification process involving zonal centrifugation in which the nonviral antigens are separated from the virus particles. The effectiveness of these inactivated influenza vaccines has been difficult to evaluate, but the immunity induced seems to be short-lived (about 4 months). Live virus vaccines appear to induce a more effective and long-lasting immunity against disease by virulent viruses. The Russians have used live influenza vaccines for many years. Currently several types of influenza vaccines are being developed in the United States.

The first approach involves the development of temperature-sensitive (ts) mutants of the influenza subtypes by Chanock, Murphy and associates. The temperature of the upper respiratory tract is 32–34° C while that of the lower respiratory tract is 37° C. The virulent forms of the influenza virus replicate between 30–40° C. Since ts mutants of the influenza virus subtypes are unable to grow at 37° C, it was reasoned that ts mutants might produce only a mild infection of the upper but not lower respiratory tract, yet also induce immune resistance. This reasoning has been supported by the observations that a ts mutant of the Hong Kong A_3 virus (ts-1-E) was unable to function at 38° C, was able to infect all human volunteers into which it was intranasally inoculated, induced mild respiratory tract symptoms in less than 25% of those inoculated, and stimulated high concentrations of secretory antibody in the respiratory tract and moderate concentrations of humoral antibody. When these vaccinated volunteers were subsequently exposed to the wild type (virulent) virus, they were protected from influenza. Since the ts-1-E mutant is stable (i.e., does not revert to the virulent wild type virus) and is not transmissible, it is considered safe for use in young children and elderly individuals. Davenport, Maassab and colleagues have, by recombination, transferred the ability to replicate efficiently at 25° C but not above 41° C to current A_3 influenza virus variants. The cold-adapted influenza variant was able to stimulate both secretory and humoral antibodies in 1,200 human volunteers inoculated intranasally without causing symptoms of influenza. This cold-adapted influenza variant is also stable and not transmitted under natural conditions.

Kilbourne advocates vaccinating against the influenza virus neuraminidase followed by either a natural or planned infection by the wild type, virulent influenza virus subtype. He calls this process "infection-permissive" immunization. Antibody directed against the viral neuraminidase appears to limit the extent of influenza epidemics by inhibiting the dissemination of virus within the host. Kasel and associates have indicated that antibody to influenza virus neuraminidase may function in reducing total virus replication in tissue culture neutralization tests by inhibiting the release of virus, thereby contributing an additive effect to that of the antihemagglutinin. To accomplish his goal, Kilbourne recombined the prevailing human A_3 influenza variant with an equine influenza subtype whose hemagglutinin moiety was unrelated to that of the wild type A_3 virus. Through selective recombination, a hybrid virus was developed with the neuraminidase surface antigen "spikes" of the A_3 wild type virus but with hemagglutinin antigen "spikes" of the "irrelevant" equine influenza subtype. The hybrid, inactivated with formalin, is injected parenterally. Those injected should develop antibodies to both antigens but only the anti-A_3 neuraminidase type of antibody specificity would modify subsequent infection by virulent A_3 influenza virus.

As discussed in Chapter 8, influenza viruses possess the ability to undergo antigenic changes in either or both neuraminidase and hemagglutinin antigens. Such variation is a reflection of the full expression of the segmented viral RNA genetic information. French scientists (Hannoun and colleagues) have apparently forced an acceleration of the mutations of an A_3 variant by mimicking the natural environment in which point mutations in the viral antigens might occur. To accomplish this, they cultured the variant in the presence of specific antibodies and isolated a variant with increased resistance to the antibodies. The new variant was then cultured in the presence of antibodies specific for it. These cycles of growth and mutation were repeated until a variant was isolated that no longer mutated under these experimental conditions. This final variant is postulated as representing the endpoint of evolution within the A_3 influenza subtype. In reviewing these experiments, Maugh cites that this endpoint A_3 mutant might be expected to appear in the human population in the late 1970's. Support for this contention comes from the fact that the London 1972 influenza variant is antigenically like the first mutant that Hannoun produced in the laboratory in the preceding year.

Bacterial Vaccines

The only living bacterial vaccine available for human use is BCG (bacillus Calmette-Guérin), an attenuated bovine strain of *M. tuberculosis*. BCG is not widely used in the United States and is only recommended for use in high-risk tuberculosis situations, e.g., medical personnel in sanitariums and children living in areas of high tuberculosis prevalence. The use of BCG vaccine in high-risk areas of tuberculosis in other areas of the world has proved beneficial in protection against tuberculosis. Those immunized with BCG either failed to develop tuberculosis or developed a mild infection which was readily treated. Resistance to widespread use of BCG vaccine in the United States reflects, in part, (1) the fact that individuals with debilitating lung disease such as silicosis develop a BCG infection as severe as tuberculosis, (2) the likelihood that those with impaired cell-mediated immune responses would develop a fulminating BCG infection, and (3) the apprehension that widespread use of BCG would render the tuberculin skin test useless for the detection of tuberculosis. The widespread use of BCG vaccine in Scandinavia does not seem to have caused such problems. One BCG vaccine currently in use is a lyophilized product prepared from a dextran-glucose medium.

Immunogenic extracts containing either ribosomal or RNA-protein subfractions of the tubercle bacillus, other facultative intracellular parasites (*Salmonella typhimurium* and *Histoplasma capsulatum*) and even extracellular bacterial parasites are able to stimulate effective host resistance in mice to subsequent infection by the specific virulent microbial pathogen. If effective in humans, such immunogenic extracts of the tubercle bacillus may not invalidate the usefulness of the tuberculin skin test since the extracts appear not to stimulate tuberculin sensitivity in mice. The facultative intracellular microbial parasites are an intriguing group of pathogens in that they display no single definable virulence factor other than the survivorship of the virulent microorganisms within host macrophages. For example, rough avirulent brucellae are readily destroyed by host phagocytes while the smooth virulent brucellae take up residence within the mononuclear phagocyte. This aspect of their parasitism has confounded the development of efficient vaccines or immunogens to protect against infection by the virulent agent. In cattle, strain 19 of *Brucella abortus,* a living agent, is efficient in inducing resistance to brucellosis but is virulent in pregnant animals or when injected accidentally into man. The degree of attenuation in virulence of a bacterial vaccine obviously depends, in part, on host factors.

The usual manner for preparing killed bacterial vaccines involves the culturing of the bacteria in a suitable broth medium from which the bacteria are removed by filtration. The bacteria are then washed to remove medium ingredients, suspended in saline and killed by the addition of formalin or phenol or by ultraviolet light. *Killed* bacterial vaccines are available for cholera (*Vibrio cholerae*), whooping cough (pertussis vaccine, *B. pertussis*), plague (*Y. pestis*), typhoid fever* (*Salmonella typhosa*) and paratyphoid fevers (*Salmonella paratyphi* and *Salmonella schottmuelleri*). Various yolk sac-cultivated rickettsial vaccines are available for certain rickettsial diseases (epidemic typhus vaccine for louse-borne *Rickettsia prowazekii,* endemic [murine] typhus vaccine for flea or louse-borne *Rickettsia typhi,* and Rocky Mountain spotted fever vaccine for the tick-borne disease caused by

---

*The killed salmonella vaccines do not induce effective host resistance in adult humans to 100,000 typhoid bacilli (the infecting dose ingested in food or water), although they appear to lessen the incidence of infection in children.

Rickettsia rickettsii). A killed vaccine for *Coxiella burneti*, the causative agent of Q-fever, has been developed but is not generally available in the United States. Since the temperature and time of pasteurization of milk was raised slightly from the thermal death time of *M. tuberculosis* to that for *C. burneti*, little need for this vaccine exists. Control of the insect vectors of the other rickettsial diseases by the use of insecticides and hygienic practices has limited the need for widespread use of the typhus vaccines in the United States.

TOXOIDS.—Formalin inactivates the toxigenicity of proteinaceous bacterial exotoxins without affecting their immunogenicity. Toxins detoxified in this manner are referred to as *toxoids*. Toxoids prepared from the toxins of *C. diphtheriae* (diphtheria toxoid) and *C. tetani* (tetanus toxoid) are used routinely to immunize children.

ANTITOXINS AND ANTISERA.—For emergency use in protecting unimmunized humans against the threat of irreversible damage and death by bacterial exotoxins, antitoxins are available against diphtheria toxin, tetanus toxin, the gas gangrene toxins (toxins of *C. perfringes, C. septicum, C. oedematiens, C. bifermentans* and *C. histolyticum* in varying combinations) and against the various toxins of *C. botulinum,* (e.g., antitoxin A, antitoxin B, antitoxin C, antitoxin D and antitoxin E). These antitoxins are prepared in animals such as horses or cows, but recently human antitetanus serum has become available. Human serum or plasma containing antitoxin is a safer biologic product to use in humans since the likelihood of inducing serum sickness in the recipient is minimized. Commercial preparations of combinations of tetanus toxoid (to induce active immunization) and tetanus antitoxin (to confer passive protection) are available. These are referred to as TAT (toxoid-antitoxin) preparations.

Commercial antisera prepared in animals against rabies virus (e.g., horse antirabies serum) and anti-*Hemophilus influenza* type B serum prepared in rabbits are available for human use. The latter antiserum is used as therapy in the rare cases in which drug resistant *H. influenzae* induces meningitis.

The gamma globulin fraction prepared from pools of human sera usually contains a variety of antibodies against infectious disease agents, e.g., whooping cough, tetanus, measles, mumps, polio, chicken pox, etc. Such preparations are available for use in humans as are gamma globulin fractions prepared from human volunteers recently recovered from a specific infectious disease (convalescent serum) or who have been willingly immunized (hyperimmune serum). Preparations of immune human gamma globulin are administered prior to or during the incubation period of polio, chicken pox, rubella, infectious hepatitis or diphtheria. If administered after the appearance of symptoms, the severity of the disease may be lessened.

POLYSACCHARIDE VACCINES.—Prior to the widespread use of antibiotics, type-specific pneumococcal capsular polysaccharides (specific soluble substance, SSS) were used in humans. Currently, polysaccharide antigens prepared from *Neisseria meningitidis* serogroups A and C are being used in human volunteers. Both types of meningococcal polysaccharides stimulate antibody formation in humans. Group C polysaccharide vaccines were effective in preventing group C meningococcal disease in military recruits.

AUTOGENOUS VACCINES.—The bacteria used in autogenous vaccines are isolated from the lesions of infected individuals, cultured in broth, and prepared for injection as a killed vaccine for use in individuals from whom the microorganisms were isolated. Toxoids may also be prepared from the bacteria and used in the same manner. Autogenous vaccines are used in treating infections which are difficult to clear by antibiotic treatment, e.g., skin infections caused by pyogenic staphylococci.

COMBINED VACCINES.—Vaccines containing mixtures of various common respiratory microorganisms (bacteria and viruses) are available for use in the treatment of children with recurrent respiratory and nasopharyngeal infections.

VACCINATION REGIMENS AND CONSIDERATIONS

In Table 12–1 are listed recommended schedules for actively immunizing children against certain microbial agents. The toxoids are available in plain solution (fluid vaccine) or adsorbed to either aluminum hydroxide or aluminum phosphate (alum-precipitated toxoids). The latter type of toxoid preparation stimulates higher and more prolonged serum antibody levels with fewer injections than do the fluid toxoids. In infants and young children, diphtheria and tetanus toxoids are frequently administered along with pertussis vaccine (DPT vaccine). The pertussis vaccine is an excellent immunogen and also exerts adjuvant action.

Even though poliovirus has been demonstrated to immunosuppress T cell blastogenesis in vitro, little likelihood exists that it immunosuppresses immune responses to the DPT vaccine when both vaccination procedures are performed at the same time. The DPT vaccine is administered parenterally while the polio vaccine is given orally. By

TABLE 12-1.—RECOMMENDED SCHEDULE FOR ACTIVE IMMUNIZATION AND TUBERCULIN TESTING OF NORMAL INFANTS AND CHILDREN*†

AGE	DISEASE	IMMUNIZING MATERIAL‡
2 months	Diphtheria, pertussis, tetanus	Diphtheria and tetanus toxoids, pertussis vaccine (DPT)
	Poliomyelitis	Trivalent oral polio vaccine (OPV)
3 months	Diphtheria, pertussis, tetanus	DPT
4 months	Diphtheria, pertussis, tetanus, poliomyelitis	DPT, OPV
6 months	Poliomyelitis	OPV
12 months	Tuberculosis	Tuberculin test
	Mumps	Live mumps vaccine
	Measles	Live measles vaccine
15–18 months	Diphtheria, pertussis, tetanus, poliomyelitis	DPT, OPV
4–6 years	Diphtheria, pertussis, tetanus, poliomyelitis	DPT, OPV
12–14 years	Tetanus, diphtheria	Tetanus and adult (low dose) diphtheria toxoids (Td)
ADDITIONAL RECOMMENDATIONS		
Nonimmune children approaching puberty	Mumps	Live mumps vaccine
	Rubella	Live rubella vaccine
Children between age 1 and puberty	Diphtheria	Td
Every 10 years after childhood immunization completed	Tetanus	

*Routine vaccination against smallpox is no longer recommended.
†Adapted from the recommendation of The American Academy of Pediatrics, January, 1972. Updated July 1974 through courtesy of M. M. Carruthers, M.D.
‡Measles and rubella, mumps and rubella, and measles, mumps and rubella are available as combined vaccines.

the time that the polioviruses have replicated in the gut and disseminated, the DPT antigens have already triggered specific immune responses. As discussed in Chapter 7, many microbial agents, viruses in particular, are immunosuppressive in vivo and in vitro. Agents which infect lymphoid tissues are likely to exert immunosuppression for brief or prolonged periods of time. Inhibition or delay of T cell responsiveness (as measured by phytohemagglutinin-induced blastogenesis of peripheral blood leukocyte preparations from afflicted individuals) occurs in vivo during rubeola, rubella, hepatitis and infectious mononucleosis infection, as well as in patients with Burkitt's lymphoma, chronic lymphocytic leukemia and Hodgkin's disease.

A temporary depression (anergy) of tuberculin sensitivity has been noted during the acute phase of mononucleosis. Individuals infected as fetuses with rubella often have impaired immune responses after birth (see Chapter 7) and may shed virus for many years. For example, the urine of a 29-year-old woman who had been congenitally infected with rubella was found to contain rubella virus. Consequently, it is neither advisable to immunize children during infection nor mix certain viral vaccines (living vaccines of immunosuppressive viruses) with any other immunogen.

The populace must be kept informed of the need to vaccinate children against polio. In 1972, 20 cases of polio occurred in the United States. Apparently, fewer children between the ages of 1 and 4 were adequately immunized against polio in 1972 than in 1964 (63% versus 88%).

Respiratory infections are still the major cause of acute illness in the United States. In children under 5 years of age, death from acute disease of the lower respiratory tract is a serious concern. Many of these infections are caused by specific respiratory viruses including respiratory syncytial (RS) virus and parainfluenza viruses types 1 and 3 and by the bacterium *M. pneumoniae.*

Glezen and Denny observed that children immunized with inactivated RS-virus vaccine experience a more severe illness than do unvaccinated children upon infection with virulent RS-virus. Currently, evaluation of the efficacy of a live RS-virus vaccine is in progress. This situation is but another example of the observation that dead virus vaccines are inefficient (and possibly more harmful) in protecting the host against invasion by virulent virus than are living attenuated virus vaccines.

It is suggested that live microbial vaccines are superior to killed vaccines in imparting protective immunity because they stimulate formation of secretory antibody at the portal of entry and possibly cell-mediated immunity. Moreover, the living attenuated virus vaccines stimulate adequate levels of serum antibodies. As discussed previously, the route of antigen injection is important. The living polio vaccine, given orally, evokes protection at the initial site of viral multiplication, the gut mucosa. Living measles vaccine administered parenterally disseminates and stimulates effective protection at the site of entry (the respiratory tract) of the virulent measles virus.

The nature of the host-parasite interaction must be well comprehended in order to construct a successful immunization procedure against disease by virulent microorganisms. The recognition that BCG and *M. leprae* are facultative intracellular parasites of the reticuloendothelial system explains the observation that BCG vaccination in Uganda elicited an 80% protection against infection by the related leprosy bacillus for more than several years. BCG induces cell-mediated immune responses leading to macrophage activation and subsequent digestion of intracellular microorganisms.

How can an effective vaccination procedure be developed to protect against infection by protozoan parasites which undergo morphologic alterations within the human host? Is it possible to vaccinate against the initial microbial form deposited in man by the mosquito? Attempts to develop a useful vaccine against malaria are in progress. What about vaccines for the ever-present venereal diseases, syphilis and gonorrhea? In spite of the fact that recovery from infection (currently accomplished by use of antibiotics) does not confer permanent immunity against these two infectious diseases, effective vaccines are being sought. Virulent gonococci (*Neisseria gonorrhoeae* T_1) possess pili which cause these cocci to adhere to leukocytes, possibly hindering their phagocytic uptake, while avirulent gonococci (e.g., T_4) lack pili and are more readily phagocytized and destroyed. Thomas and associates suggest that the T_1 cocci are not phagocytically engulfed because the overall surface tension of the sticky cocci is less than that of the phagocyte. Would immunization against an effective concentration of the virulent gonococcal pili confer long-lasting immunity?

The three-dimensional conformation of antigens as they exist on the surface of the virulent microorganism, the charge of the immunopotent groups of these antigenic mosaics, and the genetic potential of the particular host to be immunized all influence the immune response of a given individual. We would not want to be rendered readily tolerant to microbial pathogens. Weigle has offered an explanation for the fact that we are not tolerant to invading viruses and bacteria. Deaggregated protein antigens equilibrate well within the tissues inducing immunologic unresponsiveness (immune tolerance); they probably reach the lymphoid tissues in higher concentration than does the aggregated immunogenic form of the same protein. Since microorganisms including viruses are particulate, they should not equilibrate well within the tissues and consequently would induce immune responsiveness and not immune tolerance.

Biologic Manipulations of the Immune Response Suppression of Antibody Production by 7S (IgG)

The RhoGAM program involves the protection of $Rh_0(D)$-negative mothers from developing antibodies against fetal $Rh_0(D)$-positive erythrocytes. The mothers receive human gamma globulin containing $Rh_0(D)$ antibody shortly (e.g., within 72 hours) after delivery of the first $Rh_0(D)$-positive child. With the delivery of each subsequent $Rh_0(D)$-positive offspring, RhoGAM is again administered to the mother. This procedure relies upon the principle of IgG feedback suppression of specific antibody for formation (see Chapter 3). It is theorized that the high affinity anti-$Rh_0(D)$ contained in the RhoGAM is able to interact with the fetal red cells bearing $Rh_0(D)$ antigen, most of which enter the mother's circulation during delivery. The antibody binding to these $Rh_0(D)$ cells prevents their being processed immunologically and promotes their disposal by phagocytes. Consequently, the mother fails to make antibody to the $Rh_0(D)$ antigen and her next offspring is no more likely to develop erythroblastosis fetalis (see Chapter 2) than was her first child. In this type of immunosuppression, the Fc portions of the 7S antibody molecules bind to the surface of macrophages; the Fab portions of the molecule are able to capture specific antigen efficiently. Support for this concept comes from the fact that only intact 7S antibody was immunosuppressive in a spleen cell culture system; $F(ab')_2$ fragments which lack Fc regions were not immunosuppressive. Presumably, the fate of such captured antigen would be subsequent ingestion and digestion by the cells, leaving the lymphocytes of the immune system unstimulated by antigen.

DESENSITIZATION

Abolishing an already established immune response is difficult and often not possible. With our present understanding of the two limbs of the immune response and both T and B memory cells, an appreciation of this difficulty exists. The use of radiolabeled antigen to seek out and destroy antigen-reactive T and B lymphocytes (T and B cell antigen-induced suicide, see Chapter 7) has been used successfully in animal experimentation, but is neither safe nor practical for human use.

"Desensitization therapy" of sensitized humans has been used for many years in the treatment of IgE-mediated immediate hypersensitivities. Following injections of diluted allergen over a period of time, certain patients have experienced a decrease in the severity of allergic symptoms. Recent evaluations of this procedure to desensitize humans allergic to ragweed have shown that it seems to be of questionable benefit. The rationale behind this therapy was to stimulate an antibody (IgG) which blocked the effect of the antibody (IgE) mediating the allergic symptoms. Since the IgE is, for the most part, bound to mast cells throughout the tissues and mucous membranes, it would seem to have an opportunity equal to, if not greater than, available IgG molecules to bind antigen. Perhaps this is the reason that prolonged desensitization injections with allergenic extracts generally seem to allay but not to abolish the allergic systems. Also, we do not know whether IgG antibody of a given antigen specificity exerts any suppression at all on the production of IgE antibody of the same specificity.

Desensitization of animals that elicit marked delayed type hypersensitive skin test responses has been accomplished with great difficulty by injecting them with large amounts of antigen. However, this desensitization of skin test reactivity is short-lived. Humans with certain diseases which affect the T cell system, e.g., sarcoidosis or Hodgkin's disease, will become anergic (lose reactivity) to skin test antigens to which they were previously reactive. Also, individuals overwhelmed by tuberculosis often will exhibit anergy upon skin testing with tuberculin.

Transfusions

When whole blood is transfused from one person to another, the likelihood that the recipient will respond immunologically to a donor antigen is high. Unless donor and recipient are identical twins, it is improbable that they contain *all the same* erythrocyte blood group antigens, HL-A and other tissue antigens, and serum antigens such as Gm allotypes and kappa chain InV antigens. Erythrocytes well matched antigenically and washed free of other cells and serum components are preferred for transfusions. The molecular mosaic of antigens that each individual displays must be appreciated and considered for a safe transfusion.

"Transfusion" of Passive Immunity

The administration of human serum (or gamma globulin) containing antibody is used routinely in the treatment of agammaglobulinemic humans as are antibiotics. Many agammaglobulinemic humans are able to make some antibody (but at low inefficient levels). Consequently, care must be taken to administer deaggregated gamma globulin to such individuals to minimize the possibility of their immunizing to globulin allotypes different from their own.

In the successful restoration of immunocompetency in immunodeficient children with lymphoid cell populations, expertise is required. This type of treatment is not routine and is currently performed at only a few medical centers where knowledgeable teams of medical and laboratory personnel are equipped to conduct the cell transplants and carefully monitor the progress of the patient. To reduce the danger of a fatal graft-versus-host (GVH) reaction in recipients following transplantation of immunocompetent stem cells (e.g., fetal thymus, fetal liver or bone marrow), it has become apparent that the major histocompatibility antigens of donor and recipient must match. A small number of children matched with histocompatible donor tissue have been immunologically reconstituted and have subsequently undergone only mild GVH reactions. Presumably, these reactions were directed against antigens other than the major histocompatibility antigens. The immunosuppressive regimen used in the treatment of a GVH reaction would also destroy donor cells. In this situation when only mild GVH reactions occur, treatment with immunosuppressive agents is withheld; the patient may recover with the grafted lymphoid cells intact and functioning. In male children who have received lymphoid cells from a sister, all functioning immunocompetent peripheral lymphocytes bear the female donor karyotype. When bone marrow cells were used as the stem cell source, several recipients subsequently became red cell chimeras bearing both their own and their sibling's major blood group antigens. A few children with dual system immune deficiencies have been reconstituted immunologically following receipt of sibling bone marrow (B cell source) and peripheral blood lymphocytes (T cell source); several children with DiGeorge's syndrome have been immunologically reconstituted following transplant of fetal thymus.

Bach and associates were able to reconstitute immunologically a male child with Wiskott-Aldrich syndrome. Since this immunodeficiency involves both a deficiency in the processing of polysaccharide antigens as well as progressive loss of cell-mediated immune responses, immunologic reconstitution was more difficult. These investigators based their therapeutic approach on information gathered from animal experiments in which immunologic reconstitutions across certain histocompatibility barriers were accomplished following destruction of recipient's antigen-reactive cells with radiolabeled antigen prior to transplant. The male Wiskott-Aldrich patient was well matched but not identically matched with his donor sister's HL-A antigens. Moreover, his erythrocytes were blood group A while hers were blood group O. In an attempt to prevent the patient's immune system from recognizing disparities in his sister's histocompatibility antigens, the following procedure was used. The recipient was first injected with a small amount of his sister's bone marrow cells. His immune system was given time to interact with his sister's unmatched antigens prior to the injection of a massive dose of cyclophosphamide. Presumably, this cytotoxic drug selectively destroyed the patient's antigen-reactive cells, i.e., those lymphocytes in the process of interacting with donor cells. Then, the boy received a bone marrow transplant from the same sister and was successfully restored to an immunologically "normal" state. All of his functioning lymphoid cells bear only the female karyotype as do his replicative bone marrow cells; his circulating erythrocytes carry both his A and the sister's O blood group antigens.

Both Lawrence-type dialyzable transfer factors and thymosin have been used successfully in a limited number of humans in the restoration of several immune deficiency states and in the control of a few metastasizing malignancies.

EXPERIMENTAL MANIPULATIONS OF IMMUNE RESPONSE

Antilymphocyte Sera

In both animals and man, antilymphocyte serum (ALS) or antilymphocyte globulin (ALG) has been used to suppress allograft rejection. ALS exerts its immunosuppressive effect on the available circulating T cells. Consequently, the induction of new T cell responses seems more readily suppressed than does the induction of B cell responses. Established antibody responses, for the most part, seem not to be abolished by ALS. Antisera to specific T cell antigens, e.g., anti-theta antigen, have been used in mice to destroy most, but not all, functioning T cells.

Hazards exist in using such immunosuppressive agents in humans. Prolonged immunosuppression by either ALS or cytotoxic drugs in transplant patients contributes to a higher incidence of malignant disease presumably through deficiencies in the T cell surveillance mechanisms. Effective cytotoxic ALS preparations are made only in a widely divergent host species (e.g., horse anti-human lymphocyte serum). The continued use of such foreign proteins in humans seems unwise.

Using Antigen as a Specific Probe and Cytotoxic Agents for Destruction of Antigen-Reactive Cells to Prevent Sensitization

The exploitation of the antigen specificity of the immune response may eventually lead to useful methods of control of the prevention of unwanted immune responses. Bach and associates used this principle in the successful treatment of the Wiskott-Aldrich syndrome previously described. Rowley and co-workers have also used the same principle in the maintenance of long-term renal transplants in rats across strong histocompatibility barriers. Specific ALG was prepared against donor rat lymphocyte antigens. The recipient rats received 10^8 donor lymphocytes 1 day before renal transplantation and specific ALG was given for a short period (about 5 days) thereafter starting on the day of transplant. Subsequently, the recipient rats lived out a normal life span carrying kidney bearing antigens markedly different from their own. *Presumably,* the first injection of foreign antigen had been distributed throughout the recipient, had interacted with antigen-reactive cells which were then destroyed in some manner by ALG directed against the donor lymphoid cells. This mechanism is merely conjectural and not proved.

Nonspecific Macrophage Activation

As discussed in Chapter 7, activation of reticuloendothelial system phagocytes by unrelated antigens has been used to treat leprosy. Following the administration of repeated injections of allogeneic (unmatched) leukocytes to lepromatous leprosy patients, skin lesions were observed to diminish; the patients appeared in better control of the infection. The effector mechanism is presumably the nonspecific activation of macrophages by lymphokines released from the interaction of activated recipient T cells with foreign antigens (allogeneic leukocytes).

Use of Bacterial Products Against Malignant Disease

For a time Coley's toxins, culture extracts containing bacterial products, were used in the treatment of malignant disease with certain beneficial results. This mode of treatment fell into disuse with the advent of chemotherapy and radiation therapy. However, interest in the use of Coley's toxins and other bacteria in the treatment of malignant disease has been revived. It is unclear whether Coley's toxins reduce selectively the number of tumor cells, or markedly alter tumor cell antigens so that they are rapidly recognized and destroyed immunologically, or merely act as immunologic adjuvants. Currently, most investigators believe that both Coley's toxins and BCG exert nonspecific actions (adjuvant effect and/or macrophage activation) against the tumor.

PHYSICAL AND CHEMICAL MANIPULATIONS OF THE IMMUNE RESPONSE

Physical Immunosuppressive Agents (X-Irradiation)

The immunologically uncommited small lymphocyte is considered to be one of the most radiosensitive cells within the body, but becomes much more radioresistant subsequent to contact with antigen. Because of this, Schwartz suggests that x-irradiation is immunosuppressive of antibody production if administered prior to antigen injection, while the same quantity of irradiation given after antigen exerts little, if any, immunosuppression. Cell-mediated immune responses such as delayed hypersensitivity are relatively resistant to x-irradiation.

Chemical Immunosuppressive Agents

ANTIHISTAMINES.—The molecular mediation of IgE-mediated injury is well understood biochemically because of the investigations of Austen and associates. Histamine, slow-reacting substance (SRS-A) and eosinophil chemotactic factor (ECF-A) are released from the lungs of asthmatics and from nasal polyps of ragweed-sensitive atopic patients upon challenge with specific allergen. Dibutyl cyclic adenosine 3',5'-monophosphate and isoproterenol (a beta adrenergic agent) induce dose-dependent suppression of IgE-mediated release of these mediator substances. Similarly, cholera toxin suppresses the release of these mediators by increasing the tissue concentration of cyclic adenosine monophosphate (cAMP). Conversely, the antigen-induced release of these mediators appears to be enhanced by alpha adrenergic stimulation (e.g., phenylephrine + propranolol and cholinergic stimulation + carbachol). SRS-A is released in greater amounts than is histamine in the lungs, while much more histamine than SRS-A is released from human nasal polyps. Antihistamines are considerably more effective in controlling the symptoms of allergic rhinitis than in the treatment of asthma.

Disodium cromoglycate (DSCG) is useful in certain types of asthmatic attacks of either allergic or nonallergic origin. Orr suggests that DSCG is not a bronchodilator or an antagonist of either histamine or SRS-A, but is an inhibitor of migration of mast cell granules to the cell's exterior, i.e., an inhibitor of mast cell degranulation.

STEROIDS.—Corticosteroids are lymphocytolytic in some species (rats and mice) but not in others (humans, monkeys and guinea pigs).

Immunosuppression by steroids alone has not yet been convincingly demonstrated in the human species. However, the anti-inflammatory effect of corticosteroids in the human appears to be well documented. The anti-inflammatory effects may be due to (1) the stabilization of lysosomal membranes with subsequent decrease in cytotoxic damage and disruption of polymorphonuclear neutrophils, and (2) the effect on the macrophage effector cell in cell-mediated immunity, wherein the MIF lymphokine is released from sensitized T cells in the presence of specific antigen and cortisol, but the released MIF is unable to inhibit the migration of macrophages in the presence of cortisol. There have been reports that corticosteroids inhibit the binding of complement to antigen-antibody complexes. Also, corticosteroids have stopped the immunocytolysis of erythrocytes in some patients even though their red cells continued to be coated with antibody. Do corticosteroids exhibit preferential binding to carbohydrate or glycoprotein receptors of cell membranes (lysosomes, macrophages and polymorphonuclear neutrophils) and of immunoglobulin complement-binding sites?

Corticosteroids are used in the treatment of immune complex-mediated injury, immune cytolysis, certain delayed hypersensitivity reactions (poison ivy) and even in prolonged anaphylactic-type injury. In combination with cytotoxic drugs, corticosteroids are of benefit in the treatment of certain lymphomas. The malignant human lymphocyte, in contrast to its normal counterpart, may either bind more corticosteroid and/or be more sensitive to its action.

CYTOTOXIC CHEMOTHERAPEUTIC
IMMUNOSUPPRESSIVE AGENTS

The immunosuppressive drugs were originally used as cancer chemotherapeutic agents and many still are. Most of the definitive studies of drug-induced immunosuppression have been carried out in animal models. It appears that the closer the drug dosage approaches the range of toxicity the greater its immunosuppressive effect. With optimal timing and manipulation of drug dosage it has been possible in animals to (1) prevent primary or secondary antibody responses, (2) induce immunologic tolerance, (3) suppress IgG formation while prolonging the production of IgM, (4) augment antibody formation or (5) suppress allograft rejection and new or established delayed hypersensitivity reactions. As yet, all of the useful immunosuppressive agents effective in blocking antibody formation are most effective if administered before the small lymphocyte is stimulated by antigen. Once antibody formation has started, larger, generally toxic amounts of

TABLE 12-2.—COMMONLY USED IMMUNOSUPPRESSANT CYTOTOXIC DRUGS

ANTIMETABOLITES*	ACTIONS†
Purine antagonists 6-mercaptopurine (6-MP), and 6-MP + imidazole ring (azathioprine, Imuran)	Blocks differentiation of small lymphocyte to large antigen-stimulated (pyroninophilic) cell. Small dose impairs CMI; moderate dose impairs CMI and IgG responses; large dose impairs CMI, IgG and IgM responses.
Folic acid antagonist Methotrexate	Blocks development of large pyroninophilic cells into small (effector) lymphocytes in small animals.
Alkylating agent‡ Cyclophosphamide (a nitrogen mustard)	Extremely active and potent in blocking differentiation of uncommitted small lymphocyte to large pyroninophilic cell.

*Azaserine, a glutamine antagonist, is also used as an immunosuppressant.
†CMI: cell-mediated immunity.
‡Includes chlorambucil, triethylenethiophosphoramide (thio-TEPA) and busulfan.

215

the drugs are necessary to interfere with antibody production. Similarly, the secondary antibody response is considerably more resistant to drug suppression than is the initial antibody response. In the drug-induced suppression of the primary antibody response, if the drug administration ceases before complete catabolism of antigen, then antibody will form. It is easier to prevent the establishment of a new delayed hypersensitivity response than to suppress an established delayed response. At times, good clinical responses are obtained without using myelotoxic levels of drugs. It is clear that all of the modes of action and side-effects of these agents on the human body remain obscure. Prolonged immunosuppression is not always required for good clinical effects and profound immunosuppression is neither desirable nor always beneficial. Some of the cytotoxic agents used to treat humans with autoimmune disease are listed in Table 12–2. In the drug treatment of autoimmune diseases, corticosteroids are usually used first. For many patients the steroid drugs alone are used in management of the disease. However, some patients with autoimmune disease appear not to benefit from steroids alone but do experience benefit from steroids used in combination with immunosuppressive drugs. As yet, little convincing evidence has been accumulated to indicate that immunosuppressive therapy of autoimmune states increases the incidence of malignancy. Skinner and Schwartz have urged a moratorium on the publication of case reports describing the treatment of single cases of SLE and recommend that subsequent investigations contain a uniform series of patients and consist of well-designed therapeutic trials. More information concerning the use of immunosuppressive agents in the long-term treatment of autoimmune diseases is needed. Most of these agents have not been available for such use until recent years.

SUGGESTED READINGS

Abrahams, S., Phillips, R. A., and Miller, R. G.: Inhibition of the immune response by 7S antibody, mechanism and site of action, J. Exp. Med. 137:870, 1973.

Bach, F. H., *et al.*: Bone marrow transplantation in a patient with Wiskott-Aldrich syndrome, Lancet 2:1364, 1968.

Brandt, B. L., Artenstein, M. S., and Smith, C. D.: Antibody responses to meningococcal polysaccharide vaccines, Infect. Immun. 8:590, 1973.

Brown, J. A. K., Stone, M. M., and Sutherland, I.: BCG vaccination of children against leprosy: First results of a trial in Uganda, Br. Med. J. 1:7, 1966.

Chiller, J. M., and Weigle, W. O.: Cellular bases of immunological unresponsiveness, Contemp. Top. Immunobiol. 1:119, 1972.

Coley, W. B.: Cited by Old, L. J., and Boyse, E. A.: *Current Enigmas in Cancer Research,* The Harvey Lectures, Series 67 (New York: Academic Press, 1973).

Farnsworth, N. R.: Immunizing biologicals, Tile and Till 56:3; 20; 52 and 62, 1970.

Freda, V. J.: The Control of Rh Disease, in Good, R. A., and Fisher, D. W. (eds.): *Immunobiology* (Stamford, Conn.: Sinauer Associates, Inc., 1971), p. 266.

Glezen, W. P., and Denner, F. W.: Epidemiology of acute lower respiratory disease in children, N. Engl. J. Med. 288:498, 1973.

Haider, S., Coutinho, M. de L., and Emond, R. T. D.: Tuberculin anergy and infectious mononucleosis, Lancet 2:74, 1973.

Harris, J. E., and Sinkovics, J. G.: Suppression of Human Immune Response, in *The Immunology of Malignant Disease* (St. Louis: The C. V. Mosby Co., 1970), p. 176.

Hornick, R. B., *et al.*: Typhoid fever: Pathogenesis and immunologic control, N. Engl. J. Med. 283:739, 1970.

Howard, J. G.: Immunological Tolerance and Immunosuppression, in Porter, R. R. (ed.): *Biochemistry,* series 1, Vol. 10, Defense and Recognition (London: Butterworths, 1973).

Kaliner, M., Wasserman, S. I., and Austen, K. F.: Immunologic release of chemical mediators from human nasal polyps, N. Engl. J. Med. 289:277, 1973.

Kasel, J. A., *et al.*: Effect of influenza anti-neuraminidase antibody on virus neutralization, Infect. Immun. 8:130, 1973.

Kempe, C. H.: To Vaccinate or Not? in Good, R. A., and Fisher, D. W. (eds.): *Immunobiology* (Stamford, Conn.: Sinauer Associates, Inc., 1971).

Lance, E. M., Medawar, P. B., and Taub, R. N.: Antilymphocyte serum, Adv. Immunol. 17:2, 1973.

Lawrence, H. S.: Transfer factor, Adv. Immunol. 11:195, 1969.

Maugh, T. H., II: Influenza (II): A persistent disease may yield to new vaccines, Science 180:1159, 1973.

Menser, M. A., *et al.*: Rubella viruria in a 29-year-old woman with congenital rubella, Lancet 2:797, 1971.

Miller, M. E.: Uses and abuses of gamma globulin, in Good, R. A., and Fisher, D. W. (eds.): *Immunobiology* (Stamford, Conn.: Sinauer Associates, Inc., 1971).

Orr, T. S. C.: Current review: Mode of action of disodium cromoglycate, Cur. Titles in Immunol. Transplant., Allergy 1:217, 1973.

Pross, H. F., and Eidinger, D.: Antigenic competition: A review of nonspecific antigen-induced suppression, Adv. Immunol. 18:133, 1974.

Rietschel, E. T.: Pyrogenicity and immunogenicity of lipid A complexed with bovine serum albumin or human serum albumin, Infect. Immun. 8:173, 1973.

Rowley, D. A., *et al.*: Specific suppression of cell-mediated immune responses, Transplant. Proc. I:580, 1969.

Santos, G. W.: Application of marrow grafts in human disease: Its problems and potential, Contemp. Top. Immunobiol. 1:143, 1972.

Schwartz, R. (ed.): Proceedings of the symposium on immunosuppressive drugs, Fed. Proc. 26:879, 1967.

Schwartz, R. S.: Therapeutic strategy in clinical immunology, N. Engl. J. Med. 280:367, 1969.

Sela, M.: *Antigen Design and the Immune Response,* The Harvey Lectures, Series 67 (New York: Academic Press, 1973), p. 213.

Skinner, M. D., and Schwartz, R. S.: Immunosuppressive therapy, N. Engl. J. Med. 287:221 and 281, 1972.

Smith, R. T.: Possibilities and problems of immunologic intervention in cancer, N. Engl. J. Med. 287:439, 1972.

Stuart, F. P., Fitch, F. W., and Rowley, D. A.: Specific suppression of renal allograft rejection by treatment with antigen and antibody, Transplant. Proc. II:483, 1970.

Thomas, D. W., Hill, J. C., and Tyeryar, F. J., Jr.: Interaction of gonococci with phagocytic leukocytes from men and mice, Infect. Immun. 8:98, 1973.

Weston, W. L., Claman, H. N., and Krueger, G. G.: Sites of action of cortisol in cellular immunity, J. Immunol. 110:880, 1973.

Index

A

Ablastin, 150
ABO antigens, 28–29
Adenosine deaminase deficiency, 127
Adjuvants, 13, 22–23
Adoptive transfer, 12, 104
Affinity, 55
Agammaglobulinemia: lymphopenic, 126
Agglutination reactions, 80, 94–96
  mixed cell, 97
Aggressin activity, 1
Allergen, 156
Alloantigens, 24, 27–35
Allograft
  definition, 31
  fetus as, 192–193
  immunity, 187–196
  tissues, host reactions to, 188–190
Alpha chain disease: immunoglobulins in, 64
Anamnestic response, 48
Anaphylaxis: chemical mediators of, mechanism of antigen-mediated release of, 157
Antibody(ies)
  antigen-antibody (*see* Antigen, -antibody)
  bacteriolytic, 149
  blocking, 187
  to blood group antigens, naturally occurring, 29
  detection of, sensitivity of various methods of, 86
  enhancing, 187
  fluorescent antibody technic, 93–94
  formation, theories of, 46–48

-mediated cytotoxicity of cells, 163–164
-mediated protective immunity, 148–159
-mediated stimulation as mechanism of immune injury, 171–172
  multiplication-inhibiting, 149
  neutralizing, 149
  production, 48–55
  of 7S, biologic manipulations of immune response suppression of, 208
  responses, primary and secondary, 49
  synthesis by plasma cells, 54
  titer of, 84
  changes in, 84–85
Antigen(s), 13–36
  ABO, 28–29
  alloantigens, 24, 27–35
  -antibody binding
    characteristics of, 80
    electrostatic forces in, 81
    forces in, nature of, 80–82
    hydrogen bonds and, 81
    hydrophobic interactions in, 81–82
    Van der Waals forces in, 81
  -antibody interactions
    identification of etiologic agent, 85
    serology, in vitro, 80–98
    specificity of, 82–83
    time course, 85–87
  autoantigen, 32–33
  blood group, 27–30
    naturally occurring antibodies to, 29

219

Antigen(s), *(Cont.)*
   cell surface, normal, transformation possibilities, 34
   chemical nature of, 20–22
   competition, 24
   definition, 13
   determinants, 16–17
      binding of immunoglobulin Fab sites and, 47
   dose vs. immunization, 18–20
   drift, 152
   endogenous, 27–35
   heterogenetic, 25
   heterophil, 25
   histocompatibility, 30–32
   HL-A *(see* HL-A antigens)
   immune response and, 24–25
   immunodominant group, 16–17
   immunogenicity of, 13
   injection route, 23–24
   -liberated transfer factor, 104
   lymphocyte surface, mobility of, 121–124
   microbial, exogenous, 25–27
      of gram-negative bacilli, representation of, 26
   mixed leukocyte culture, in tissue typing, 193–194
   particulate, 14
   physical state of, 20–22
   processing, chemical nature and physical state of, 20–22
   Rh, 29–30
   sensitization and, 212
   shift, 152
   -specific B and T lymphocytes, antigen-induced proliferation of, 18
   -specific T cell receptors, 104
   tissue, host responses to, 187–188
   tolerizing, 19
   tumor, 33–35
   valence of, 16–17
Antihistamines: as immunosuppressive agents, 213
Antilymphocyte sera, 211
Antisera, 203–204
Antitoxins, 203–204
Arboviruses, 2
Ataxia telangiectasia, 128

Autoantigen, 32–33
Autogenous vaccines, 204
Autograft: definition, 31
Autoimmune diseases
   classification of, 175
   possible etiologic mechanisms of, 176–177
Autoimmunity, 174–186
   drug-induced, 183
   microbial agents inducing, 177
   slow viruses and, 178–183
Avidity, 55

B

Bacteremia, 8
Bacterial products: use against cancer, 212–213
Bacterial vaccines, 201–204
Bacteriolytic antibody, 149
B cell defects, 125–126
   combined B and T cell, 126–128
Blastogenic factor, 100
Blastogenic inhibitor factor, 101
Blocking antibodies, 187
Blood group antigens, 27–30
   naturally occurring antibodies to, 29
B lymphocytes: antigen-specific antigen-induced proliferation of, 18

C

Cancer: use of bacterial products against, 212–213
Cells(s)
   B cell defects, 125–126
      combined B and T cell, 126–128
   cytotoxicity of, antibody-mediated, 163–164
   interactions and immune response, 124–125
   markers, 115–116
      (in mouse), 114–115
   -mediated immune response in vivo, 105–106
   -mediated immunity *(see* Immunity, cell-mediated)
   phagocytic cell deficiencies, 128–129

plasma, antibody synthesis by, 54
rosette-forming, and T cell receptors, 114
T (*see* T cell)
Children: recommended schedule for active immunization and tuberculin testing, 205
CMI (*see* Immunity, cell-mediated)
Commensalism, 1
Commensals, 1
Complement, 69–79
    biologic significance, 72–73
    deficiencies, 77–78
    fixation, 96
    -fixation test, 71–72
    pathway
        alternate, 73–75
        classic, activation of, 69–71
Coombs' test, 95
    indirect, 95
Coulombic forces: and antigen-antibody binding, 81
Cytolysis: immune, of erythrocytes, 160–163
Cytotoxic agents: and sensitization, 212
Cytotoxic chemotherapeutic immunosuppressive agents, 214–216
Cytotoxicity
    of cells, antibody-mediated, 163–164
    testing, 97

D

Desensitization, 208–211
Diapedesis, 10
Drug-induced autoimmunity, 183
Dysgammaglobulinemia: lymphopenic, 127

E

Electroimmunodiffusion, 93
Electrostatic forces: and antigen-antibody binding, 81
Endotoxin tolerance, 149
Enzymatic cleavage: causing immunoglobulin fragments, 41

Erythrocytes: immune cytolysis of, 160–163
Exocytosis, 50

F

Fetus: as allograft, 192–193
Fluorescent antibody technic, 93–94

G

Gamma chain disease: immunoglobulins in, 64
Genetic capacity: of immunization recipient, and immune response, 17–18
Genetic deficiency diseases: primary, 128
Glomerular injury: immunologically mediated, in systemic lupus erythematosus, 168
Graft
    allograft (*see* Allograft)
    autograft, definition, 31
    homostatic, 32
    homovital, 32
    syngeneic, definition, 31
    syngraft, definition, 31
    -vs.-host reaction, 31
        to allografted tissues, 188–190
    xenograft, definition, 31

H

Haptens, 13, 92
H chain diseases: immunoglobulins in, 63–66
Hemagglutination
    -inhibition reactions, 94
    -inhibition test, 95
    reaction, direct, 94
    test, passive, 94
Histocompatibility antigens, 30–32
HL-A antigens
    in tissue typing, 193–194
    tumor and allograft immunity and, 194
Homostatic grafts, 32
Homovital grafts, 32
Host
    barriers, 8

Host, *(Cont.)*
  defense mechanisms, 8–12
  as favorable microenvironment,
    4–7
  graft-vs.-host reaction, 31
    to allografted tissues, 188–190
  immune systems, interrelation-
    ships between oncogenesis
    and, 190–192
  immunity, protective, 148–154
    inducible nonimmunologic fac-
      tors, 150
  microorganism dissemination
    within, 8
  microorganism localization within,
    140–146
  microorganism persistence within,
    140–146
  -parasite interactions, 140–155
    introduction, 1–12
  reactions
    to allografted tissues, 188–190
    to tissue antigens, 187–188
  three host cascade systems, inter-
    relation of, 75–77
Humoral factor: thymic, 113–114
Hydrogen bonds: and antigen-
    antibody binding, 81
Hydrophobic interactions: in
    antigen-antibody binding,
    81–82

I

Idiotypes, 47
Ig *(see* Immunoglobulin)
Immune cytolysis: of erythrocytes,
    160–163
Immune deficiency *(see* Immunode-
    ficiency)
Immune deviation, 24
Immune opsonins, 142, 149
Immune precipitation reactions, 87
Immune response
  antigens and, 24–25
  biology of, 108–139
  cell-mediated, in vivo, 105–106
  cellular interactions, 124–125
  genetic capacity of immunization
    recipient and, 17–18
  immunization and, 17–20
  induction of
    macrophage in, 122–123
    monocyte in, 122–123
    two-signal model of, 119–121
  manipulations of, 197–218
    chemical, 213–214
    experimental, 211–213
    physical, 213–214
  nutrition and, 116
  ontogeny, 109–113
  phylogeny, 108–109
  suppression of antibody produc-
    tion by 7S, biologic manipu-
    lations of, 208
  transfusions and, 209
Immunity
  acquired, 11–12
    artificially, active, 12
    artificially, passive, 12
    naturally, active, 11–12
    naturally, passive, 12
  allograft, 187–196
  autoimmunity *(see* Autoimmunity)
  cell-mediated, 99–107
    induction of, 105
    skin test response, 99–102
    specific, 150–151
    transferability of, 104–105
  host, protective, 148–154
    inducible nonimmunologic fac-
      tors, 150
  innate, 11
  passive, "transfusion" of, 209–211
  protective, antibody-mediated,
    148–149
  tumor, 187–196
Immunization
  active, recommended schedule for
    normal infants and children,
    205
  immune response and, 17–20
  nonresponders, 17
  recipient, genetic capacity of, and
    immune response, 17–18
  responders, 17
  vs. antigen dose, 18–20
  vs. immunologic unresponsive-
    ness, 18–20
Immunoconglutinin, 73

Immunocytoadherence, 97
Immunodeficiency diseases, 125–133
  primary, 125–129
  secondary, 129–133
Immunodiffusion: radial, 91–92
Immunoelectrophoresis, 92
  counter, 93
  quantitative, 93
Immunogen(s), 13–36
  artificial, 14–16
  definition, 13
  natural biologic substances as,
    13–14
  synthetic, 14–16
  types of, 13–16
Immunogenicity: of antigens, defini-
    tion, 13
Immunoglobulin(s), 37–68
  abnormalities, 66
  allotypic markers of, 45–46
  in alpha chain disease, 64
  biologic functions of, 58–61
  characteristics of, 39
  Fab sites, binding of antigen de-
    terminants and, 47
  fragments due to enzymatic cleav-
    age, 41
  G
    antibody production by, biolog-
      ic manipulations of immune
      response suppression of, 208
    structural domains, diagram, 43
  G_1 molecule, basic structure of, 38
  in gamma chain disease, 64
  in H chain diseases, 63–66
  hinge region, 40
  levels, 55–58
  monomeric, 44
  in Mu chain disease, 65–66
  in myeloma, multiple, 61–63
  pathologic counterparts of, 59,
    61–66
  polymeric, 44
  properties of, 37–45
  structure of, 37–45
  in Waldenström's macroglobuline-
    mia, 63
Immunologic deficiency (see Immu-
    nodeficiency)
Immunologic injury, 156–173

  anaphylactic type, 156–160
  antibody-mediated stimulation as
    mechanism of, 171–172
  cell mediated, 169–171
  cytotoxic type, 160–164
  immune complex-mediated, 164–
    169
    mechanism of, 166–167
  mechanisms of, 156–173
  type I, 156–160
  type II, 160–164
  type III, 164–169
    mechanism of, 166–167
  type IV, 169–171
Immunologic tolerance: definition,
    18–19
Immunologic unresponsiveness: vs.
    immunization, 18–20
Immunoresponsiveness: functioning,
    116–119
Immunosupressive agents
  chemical, 213–214
  cytotoxic chemotherapeutic, 214–
    216
  physical, 213
Infants: recommended schedule for
    active immunization and tu-
    berculin testing, 205
Injury (see Immunologic injury)
Interferon, 150
Irradiation: as immunosuppressive
    agent, 213

                  K

Koch's Postulates, 7

                  L

Lawrence type dialyzable transfer
    factor, 104
Leukocyte culture antigens: mixed,
    in tissue typing, 193–194
Lupus erythematosus: systemic, im-
    munologically mediated glo-
    merular injury in, 168
Lymphocyte(s)
  antigen-specific B and T, antigen-
    induced proliferation of, 18
  receptors, and tumor and allograft
    immunity, 194

Lymphocyte(s), *(Cont.)*
surface antigens and receptors, mobility of, 121–124
surface markers, 114–116
(in mouse), 114–115
Lymphocytotoxin, 101
Lymphokines, 100
Lymphopenic agammaglobulinemia, 126
Lymphopenic dysgammaglobulinemia, 127
Lymphotoxin, 101

M

Macroglobulinemia: Waldenström's immunoglobulins in, 63
Macrophage
activating factor, 100
activation, nonspecific, 212
aggregating factor, 100
role in induction of immune response, 122–123
Malignant disease: use of bacterial products against, 212–213
Microabsorption technic, 97
Microbial agents: as inducers of autoimmunity, 177
Microbial antigens, exogenous, 25–27
of gram-negative bacilli, representation of, 26
Microbial virulence factors, 146–148
Microenvironment: favorable, host as, 4–7
B₂ Microglobulin, 194
Microorganisms
dissemination within host, 8
localization within host, 140–146
persistence within host, 140–146
MLC antigens: in tissue typing, 193–194
Monocyte: role in induction of immune response, 122–123
Mu chain disease: immunoglobulins in, 65–66
Myeloma: multiple, immunoglobulins in, 61–63

N

Neutralizing antibodies, 149
Nezelof's syndrome, 126
Nutrition: and immune response, 116

O

Oncogenesis: interrelationships between host immune systems and, 190–192
Opsonins: immune, 142, 149
Ouchterlony double diffusion, 89–90

P

Parasite-host interactions, 140–155
introduction, 1–12
Parasitism, 1
Phagocyctic cell deficiencies, 128–129
Plasma cells: antibody synthesis by, 54
Polypeptide structures: immunogenic and nonimmunogenic, 15
Polysaccharide(s)
complex, 14
vaccines, 204
Precipitation reactions: immune, 87
Precipitin
reactions, 80
test
ring, 87–88
variations of, 87–94
Proliferative inhibitory factor, 101
Proteins: serum, electrophoretic migration of, schematic representation, 37

Q

Quellung reaction, 88–89
diagrammatic representation, 89

R

Radial immunodiffusion, 91–92
Radiation: as immunosuppressive agent, 213

Radioimmunoassay technics, 93
Rh antigens, 29–30
Rosette tests, 97

S

7S: biologic manipulations of immune response suppression of antibody production by, 208
Sensitization: antigens and cytotoxic agents, 212
Septicemia, 8
Skin test response, 99–102
Steroids: as immunosuppressive agents, 213–214
Symbiosis: definition, 1
Syngeneic graft: definition, 31
Syngraft: definition, 31

T

T cell
    defects, 126
        combined B and T cell, 126–128
    function, assays of, 103
    receptors
        antigen-specific, 104
        rosette-forming cells and, 114
    system, 102–103
Telangiectasia: ataxia, 128
Thymic humoral factor, 113–114
Tissue
    allografted, host reactions to, 188–190
    antigens, host responses to, 187–188
    typing, 96
        HL-A antigens in, 193–194
        MLC antigens in, 193–194
Titer of antibodies, 84
    changes in, 84–85
T lymphocytes: antigen-specific, antigen-induced proliferation of, 18
Toxoids, 203
Transfer
    adoptive, 12, 104

factor
    antigen-liberated, 104
    Lawrence type dialyzable, 104
Transfusion
    immune response and, 209
    of passive immunity, 209–211
Tuberculin testing: of normal infants and children, recommended schedule, 205
Tumor
    antigen, 33–35
    immunity, 187–196

V

Vaccination, 197
    regimens and considerations, 204–208
Vaccines
    autogenous, 204
    bacterial, 201–204
    combined, 204
    definition, 197
    polysaccharide, 204
    types currently in use, 197–204
    virus, 197–201
Van der Walls forces: in antigen-antibody binding, 81
Viremia, 8
Virulence, 1–4
    establishment of, 7–8
    factors, microbial, 146–148
    measurement of, 7–8
Virus(es)
    arboviruses, 2
    slow, and autoimmunity, 178–183
    vaccines, 197–201

W

Waldenström's macroglobulinemia: immunoglobulins in, 63
Wiskott-Aldrich syndrome, 127–128

X

Xenograft: definition, 31
X-irradiation: as immunosuppressive agent, 213